The New Arrival

SARAH BEESON

MBE

The New Arrival

The heartwarming true story
of a 1970s trainee nurse

HARPER

HARPER

An imprint of HarperCollins*Publishers*
77–85 Fulham Palace Road
Hammersmith, London W6 8JB

www.harpercollins.co.uk

First published by HarperCollins*Publishers* 2014

A catalogue record for this book
is available from the British Library

ISBN 978-0-00-752007-7

Printed and bound in Great Britain by
Clays Ltd, St Ives plc

MIX
Paper from
responsible sources
FSC
www.fsc.org **FSC® C007454**

FSC™ is a non-profit international organisation established to promote
the responsible management of the world's forests. Products carrying the
FSC label are independently certified to assure consumers that they come
from forests that are managed to meet the social, economic and
ecological needs of present or future generations,
and other controlled sources.

Find out more about HarperCollins and the environment at
www.harpercollins.co.uk/green

Dedicated to my dear friend, mentor and colleague
Patricia Wrennall, health visitor

About Sarah Beeson

In 1969 17-year-old Sarah Beeson – then Sarah Hill – arrived in Hackney in the East End of London to begin her nursing career. Six years later she went into health visiting, practising for over 35 years in Kent and Staffordshire, building up a lifetime's expertise and stories through working with babies and families.

In 1998 Sarah received the Queen's Institute for Nursing Award. In 2006 she was awarded an MBE for Services to Children and Families by Queen Elizabeth II.

She later married and became Sarah Beeson. Now she divides her time between Staffordshire and London.

1

It was 23 September 1969, already past nine o'clock in the morning. I was still sitting alone on the back seat of my father's blue Rover P4, waiting for my mother to emerge from the house. I impatiently kicked my white round-toed calf-length Mary Quant boots against the front passenger seat. After years of practice I could do this without scuffing either the seat or my well-worn but perfectly presentable boots. All the time I kept my eyes fixed on the open front door of Uplands, our *gentleman's country residence* – I was leaving as soon as my mother deigned to join me. 'Typical,' I muttered under my breath. I took my last long sniff of sea air and slowly counted to ten. My ears pricked at the distinct click of my mother's court shoes on the parquet floor; she was finally making her way down the hall and outside. Two steps behind her was Harold, my father's driver, carrying my battered old school trunk with the initials SH fading on the side. I watched icily as Mum unnecessarily oversaw Harold loading my trunk into the boot of the car before he opened her door and she slipped effortlessly onto the seat next to me. Neither of us said anything; we both sat straight backed with our knees together on either side of the back seat – my mother's handbag resting perfectly upright between us. Harold took up his place at the wheel and I felt my heart skip with excitement as he started the engine and we finally made our way down the quarter-of-a-mile driveway.

I watched idly through the window as we sped down the narrow country lanes to meet the seashore and the grey little town below. Llanelli whizzed past me, stonewashed modest houses, mothers pushing carriage-like prams, small vans delivering to butchers and greengrocers. It seemed such a small, small world. Too small for my mother. She sat day by day in the big house waiting for my father to return – one of the bosses at Thyssen's, he arrived home almost every night of the week with at least two dinner guests expecting to be served a three-course meal. Mum rarely complained. Also at the table, merrily sitting alongside Dad's international business associates, were my older brother and sister, William and Jane, the younger two, Bridget and Stephen, and often our school chums. Both children and adults consumed vast amounts of prawn cocktail and pink champagne off the custom-made boardroom-sized dining table. Dad would say to our dinner guests, 'You've got to be quick in this house,' as his gaggle of children lapped up our grub whether it was a curry, a Chinese or a roast.

This place was too small for me too; it wasn't my home, just the latest stop after a childhood of constantly moving to new towns and villages. Dad was a top civil engineer and we moved with him; so one year he would be working on the Dartford Tunnel and we were living it up in Sevenoaks. Next we'd moved into a house custom built by my dad, on the hilltop overlooking Loch Etive, while he built the new hydroelectric plant to supply electricity for the west coast of Scotland. I wouldn't miss this house; Scotland had been the beloved place of my childhood – it was there I made the transition from little girl to brooding teenager. Today, my only pang of regret was as the car went past the Chinese takeaway belonging to my best friend Sue's family. Of course the shutters were down at that time of the morning, but still I looked for her heart-shaped face in the upstairs window. She wasn't there.

Mum folded her hands, her long fingers cocooned in spotless white gloves which rested lightly in her lap. I peeked up at her and drank in her portrait. Her slender frame and long neck were enhanced by a cream polo-neck jumper, complete with matching coat and pillbox hat. Her hair was still naturally dark, though she was over fifty, and swept up into a glossy brown bun on the back of her head. She was perfectly made up with just a dash of powder on her pretty tanned nose, a sweep of grey shadow on her sparkly eyes and a smear of pink lipstick on her mouth – just right for this time of the morning. Beside her I was a pale-skinned dwarf. When standing, she towered a good eight inches above me, more in heels, which she usually wore. Apart from my obvious lack of height compared to the rest of my family, I took more after Dad on the inside too. Put together my brothers William and Stephen were like a pair of giant bookends. My sisters Jane and Bridget were tall and graceful like Mum. But though we all got into our fair share of scrapes, I was always the one to unintentionally rile my mother or be in hot water with the nuns at boarding school, as I shared my father's sense of fun, sometimes at the expense of what we *ought* to have been doing. I wished it was just me and him driving to London on one of our rare drives together.

I heard Mum sigh as Harold deviated from the main road down yet another narrow country lane – one of his so-called shortcuts that doubled the length of the journey. 'We won't be there till sunset at this rate,' she hissed.

It was the second thing she'd said to me all morning, the first being, 'Is that what you're wearing?' I'd come down to breakfast in my red suede miniskirt and black polo-neck top. I was eager to be off and already wearing my three-quarter-length navy Reefer jacket with the brass buttons, my hair still wet and falling unfettered and uncut to my chest. I considered it a rhetorical question, and moodily helped myself to the toast, jam and a cup of tea which were all ready and waiting on the breakfast table.

Now the silence was broken Mum settled upon a topic for the journey – her incredulity at both my choice of career and location. 'All the money your father's spent on your education. You won't last two weeks.'

I didn't say anything in reply. I leaned forward and asked Harold if we could have the radio on. He tuned in to Radio

One just for me. Mum huffed and opened up her square white leather handbag and to my relief took out her knitting. I was glad to hear the friendly familiar voice of Tony Blackburn on the car radio as he introduced The Archies, and soon the sound of 'Sugar, Sugar' filled the highly polished Rover.

But my mother had made her point and I couldn't help but think back to my last year at school – my secret study in the library. I kept going back and reading up on nursing. I had been pretty appalled at the life of a nurse too, and yet I felt so drawn to it. I wanted to make a difference in the world and to help people who needed care and compassion. When my grandfather had been very sick it had been me who sat with him, comforted and cared for him, not my brothers and sisters or even my parents, who had been uncomfortable around illness. It felt to me it was the right thing to do; it felt like it was my gift to him. But even my friends hadn't thought nursing a worthwhile ambition – nice privately educated young ladies weren't meant to do that sort of thing (unless you count my heroine Florence Nightingale, of course).

It wasn't until I was summoned to the headmistress's office that I made my final decision. She informed me, 'Sarah, I've put your name down for teacher training,' something nice respectable girls could do until they had babies. I found myself replying, 'Well that's a surprise as I'm going to be a nurse,' and flouncing out of her office feeling as pleased as punch. As soon as I'd done my O-levels I went to do my

Community Voluntary Service in a children's home in Wiltshire. I knew then that nursing was my calling. I'd completed my nursing application and accepted my place without consulting anyone. I'd not told my parents or even mentioned it to my siblings. My parents were horrified at my decision – here I was, 17 years old and going to be a student nurse in Hackney in the East End of London of all places. This life was not what anybody had in mind for Sarah Elizabeth Hill.

Ours was a happy, busy family, there was always something going on – Stephen accidentally setting fire to my father's wood or the farmer's pigs getting in and eating the precious crop of strawberries – but our parents had high expectations. Bridget my roommate was sitting her exams and Stephen wasn't even a teenager, yet William was studying civil engineering at university under duress and Jane was doing fashion at art college.

Why, I asked myself, was it suddenly necessary to be driven down by Harold with my mother as escort? After all, they'd been sending me on buses, trains and planes unaccompanied to boarding school from infancy. I decided it was all down to Mum's morbid curiosity, or most likely the hope that I'd take one look at the nurses' accommodation and hot foot it back to South Wales in Dad's chauffeur-driven car. Well, if that was the plan, my parents were going to find themselves disappointed.

★ ★ ★

The car finally edged its way down bustling Homerton High Street early that afternoon. There was a constant buzz of small delivery vans and buses going up and down. The pavements and the houses were narrow and greyish and rows and rows of small shop fronts made up the face of the high street. Harold pulled into the grounds of Hackney Hospital and parked next to the large circular lawn at the front of the nurses' home. It towered above us; six storeys high of 1930s' sandy-grey brick – relentlessly flat and institutional looking. I looked up at the neatly stacked uniform windows in the plain block; I couldn't wait to know which one would belong to me.

'Is this it?' said my mother in disbelief. 'What a dreadful place; I don't think your father will like you living in this sort of neighbourhood.'

I jumped out of the car, eager to stretch my legs and find my room. Harold was already taking my trunk out of the boot. 'Just pop it in the entrance, please, Harold. I'll take it from there,' I instructed. He silently went ahead and disappeared into the building. Mum was still in the car. She wound down the window slowly. I went round to her side of the car and popped my head in. 'I'll be fine from here. You get off,' I tried to insist in what I thought was a casual but confident manner.

'No, I want to make sure you'll be all right,' she said, opening the car door as I stumbled back.

'All right,' I said, stalking off to the entrance, passing Harold on his way out of the building with my mother hot on my heels.

I pushed my way through the heavy double doors and stepped into the large whitewashed hall. It was plain, yet purposeful. Heavily curtained windows proceeded straight and tall down the length of the black-and-white tiled corridor. At the end, a staircase curved off and up into the heart of the building. I saw Harold had placed my trunk under the wooden table that stood on a faded though spotless rug in the hallway. The table, bathed in shadowy light, was made welcoming by a vase of white carnations. This was the entrance to my new life – I was home.

'It's very clean,' said my mother, running a gloved finger over the table. 'Like a hospital. Smells like one too,' she added with a twitch of distaste. She couldn't be doing with hospitals or sick people; they made her feel uncomfortable.

'You'd better get going, Mum. You want to be back in time for Harold to pick up Dad from work.'

'I thought I'd see your room, take you into town for a nice lunch. Make sure you're properly fed.'

'I'll be fine,' I insisted. I knew Mum was worried, that she was trying to be kind, but I just wanted to get on with things – I have always hated long goodbyes.

She looked into my face, searching for some hint of whether she should insist I return home with her right now. 'If only you were at a nice hospital in the West End or Grosvenor Square, near your father's head office.'

'I want to be here. I will be fine. Please don't worry.'

Mum turned and then hesitated. 'If you're sure …'

'I am,' I said, stepping forward and giving her a brief hug.

I could see Harold through the pane of glass in the big front door. The engine was running – he knew the score.

'If you're sure,' she repeated, and this time it wasn't a question. I smiled and gave her a single nod of the head as I opened the double doors for her and she walked steadfastly back to the Rover.

She paused once again as her hand reached for the door handle. I gave a little wave of encouragement from the front step of the nurses' home and to my relief Harold appeared at her elbow to open the car door and she slipped elegantly inside. 'Safe journey,' I called.

'I'll write,' she called back through the open window as the car pulled off back down the drive towards the gates. I saw her quickly winding it back up again as they found themselves once more heading towards Homerton High Street.

Back in the nurses' home I made my way gingerly down the corridor, passing cleaners sweeping and polishing, and nurses hurrying in and out; no one took any notice of me – everyone had a job to do and soon I would too. I had to head directly to Home Sister's room to report for duty. I remembered from my interview in the summer that it was just to the left of the main entrance. I almost skipped as I trotted past the half-open door of the reading room, glancing at the white caps peaking up over the tops of chintzy sofas – but I did a double take when I spotted uncovered greased-back hair looming over the tops of the armchairs. Hang on a minute – men, men are allowed in the nurses' home, I said to myself. I guessed this room wasn't really for reading and study but somewhere to meet up with your boyfriend. *NB!* I laughed quietly to myself. Just as well Mum hadn't accompanied me or I'd have never been shot of her; she hadn't put me in a convent boarding school for nothing.

Once in front of Home Sister's inner sanctum I took a deep breath and knocked on the door. I waited but there was no answer. I knocked again but still nothing. I thought I heard a noise from within, a soft shuffle and a clink. I hesitated and cast my eyes about. What was I to do? Where was I to go?

'You looking for Home Sister, pet?' I heard a voice behind me sing out down the corridor in a lyrical accent I'd never encountered before.

I turned round and saw a small nurse in a light blue dress and crisp white apron smiling at me, her hip resting against the wall. Her bright blue eyes crinkled up at the corners; she must have been at least forty. She had wild curly chestnut hair poking out from under her nurse's cap and red lipstick stained her plump little mouth. With two highly arched black eyebrows and a perfectly round blush on each of her white cheeks, she looked like a china doll. I thought make-up was forbidden.

'Yes, I was told to report to Home Sister on arrival.'

'Hill, is it?'

'Yes.'

'I'm Wade. Edie Wade. Home Sister is, shall we say, indisposed.' I looked blank. She softly chuckled and mimed taking a drink and then played the drunk wobbling about a bit and bumping into the wall. I stifled my laughter, placing my hand over my mouth. 'You should have come before lunch,' she told me.

'Oh, we didn't arrange a time.'

'You'll learn the right time soon enough. Come on, I'll show you to your room.'

'Thank you,' I replied rather meekly, my former confidence ebbing away a little at having already been shown to not know the score in front of a real nurse.

'Where are your bags?'

'My trunk is under the table in the hall.'

'Is it now? Well, I'll ask the porter to bring it up to you. You're on the fourth floor, room 17. You wouldn't want to heft it up all that way yourself. Follow me,' said Wade, tapping off down the corridor and springing up the stairs. My spirits lifted by her easy manner and dancing feet, I rushed after Wade, following her little black shoes as she did toe heel leads all the way to my room.

'I've only been here a week myself,' said Wade.

'You're a nurse already though, aren't you?'

'Not young enough to be a trainee, hey?'

'No, no, I meant …'

'I'm only teasing you, pet. I've been a nurse off and on in-between bairns ever since I left the music halls. I'm here to do my midwifery.'

'You were in the music halls?' I asked, amazed and impressed.

'Ever since I was little girl. I've done a turn with Morecambe and Wise, not to mention Julie Andrews,' she told me, belting out 'The Hills are Alive with the Sound of Music'. I looked around, embarrassed and unsure of what to say next.

Wade took a key out of her pocket and unlocked the door before handing it over. It swung open to reveal a small rectangular cell lit by a single window. I stepped into my new room; it was simply furnished, just a single bed with neatly folded sheets and blankets resting on it, waiting for me to make it, a bare wooden chest that folded out into a desk and an empty cupboard. A hand basin stood in a little recess, with a mirror and vacant shelves above it waiting to be filled with my things. Apart from that there was only a laundry box which served as a seat. I walked over, removed the lid and peeked in.

'I keep bottles of booze in mine. It's the one place Home Sister won't scout them out,' snorted Wade. I smiled broadly. My room.

'There are no plugs in here so if you want to use a hair dryer or anything you'll have to make do with the hall socket. I'm just next door,' continued Wade. 'Have you eaten?'

'No,' I replied.

'Ah, come with me then, I'll show you the nurses' dining room – it's almost tea time. Home Sister normally rallies after a good strong cup of tea.'

I obediently followed Wade. There were already dozens of nurses sitting at round tables, which were covered in white table cloths with a place neatly laid out for each girl. I walked behind Wade to the counter. My eyes met with bowlfuls of pies, mash, sausages, chips, roasted meats, curry, rice, fish, bread rolls, soup, umpteen traditional puddings, jugs of custard, and pots of tea and coffee. It was tempting stodge and I vowed not to make a habit of eating it and looked penitently at the salad bar.

'What do you fancy, Hill?' she asked.

'What are you having?'

'My regular – sausage, eggs, bacon and a fried slice of bread with a cuppa.'

'I'll have the same. How much is that?' I asked, reaching into my pocket for my purse.

'You've forgotten it's "all in". Bed and board.'

'Oh, yes of course, how silly of me.'

'Come on, we'll eat up and then try our luck and see if Home Sister is ready to receive callers. You'll need your uniform pressed and ready before you see Matron at eight o'clock tomorrow morning. I've heard you're starting on the Infants Ward. It's nice there but watch out for that Sister Nivern, she's a right devil; you do not want to get on the wrong side of her,' Wade instructed me, as she heaped sausages on to my plate for tea.

At the thought of what Sister Nivern might have in store for the new girl, I almost lost my appetite.

2

Who is this nurse in front of me, I asked of my reflection. I was standing before the mirror on the back of my wardrobe door. My neatly pressed striped blue dress fell just above the knee of my black stockings. One by one, I picked up the items of my trade that I had laid out on the desk the night before. First I adorned myself with a red, a blue and a black pen, and a pair of scissors, all lined up in a row in my top pocket. 'All present and correct,' I said to my reflection with a giggle. Dad had been an officer in the war and drilled us as children. I picked up my little upside-down nurse's watch and pinned it on the other side of my chest like a medal and briefly wondered why my father had never collected his own medals – he'd won enough. My student nurse's uniform was so much better than the school boaters and blazers I'd been forced to wear so all the children in the village knew you were posh, knew you were the boss's daughter. Here I was going to be just like everyone else, here I was going to be me; whoever that was. I slipped on my new white apron and wrapped the white belt which held it in place tightly around my waist. My eyes glanced down once again at the stiff white collar waiting on the desk. I'd already had several failed attempts to pin it on. This stupid collar is going to make me late, I huffed. I took a deep breath and picked up the collar and studs, and closing my eyes I wiggled the silly thing on. It felt itchy and scratchy against my neck but I persisted and after a bit of wincing I finally felt the studs pop into place. Thank heaven. I quickly picked up my hairbrush and made hasty strokes into my mass of long dark hair, pinning it into a neat bun. Then I slowly took up my snowy student nurse's cap and crowned myself, jabbing in more pins to keep it in place. Now for the *pièce de résistance* – my black cape. I loved this best of all and whirled it around my shoulders and gave a little twirl in front of the mirror as I watched the swish of the scarlet lining flare out around me. I was ready.

I hurried out of the nurses' home. I knew the route to Matron's office on the ground floor of the hospital; I'd prac-tised it yesterday evening so I wouldn't get lost and risk arriving flustered and late. I didn't want to blot my copy-book on the first day. I took a deep breath and knocked on Matron's door.

'Enter,' commanded a calm, low voice. Matron sat already engrossed in paperwork behind a large desk. She was wiry, her skin was pale and taut, stretched over high cheekbones and a strong forehead. The flow of her dark blue dress was only broken by the whiter than white cuffs and collar. She didn't have the softness of the other nurses in their aprons, but was formal, removed from the menial everyday tasks of care. Her hair was pinned very tightly into a bun but it waved in white, grey and chestnut strands from her high forehead to her cap. She had small ears, a hooked nose and thin lips that even now looked like she was chewing over something. She gave a flash of yellowing teeth when she looked up and saw me standing in front of her desk but then even that hint of a smile was gone.

'Hill.'

'Yes, Matron.'

'You are on time today, but according to my records,' she picked out a piece of paper from the pile she had been looking over, 'you are in fact three months early.'

'Matron?' I mumbled, panic rising from within me.

'You cannot be part of the September intake of the Nurses Training School because you neglected to realise that you have to be eighteen to train to be a nurse. You, Hill, are not eighteen, not until the twenty-third of November.'

'I didn't know that.'

'Didn't know you were underage or when your birthday is?'

'I didn't know I was underage to train. I did put my date of birth on my application, Matron.'

She glared at me. This was not the time to point out that she should have noticed she had illegally employed me. 'Well, as you are here, Hill, you can make yourself useful by helping out on the Infants Ward and join the next intake in the New Year.'

'Yes, Matron.'

She stood and held out her hand to shake mine. 'Good luck, Hill,' and I was dismissed.

I was glad to be away from Matron's office and practically hurdled up the stairs to the Infants Ward for fear of her calling me back to tell me she'd changed her mind and was sending me home till January. I eagerly took in the long parades of beds on each ward as I passed by. It was all very Florence Nightingale, all what you'd expect from a Victorian building that had been built to be a workhouse, not a hospital. It had stuck to that institutional layout of having row upon row of neatly lined-up beds stretching out before you, all well kept if a bit anonymous. So, when I boldly pushed my way through the doors to the Infants Ward, I was surprised to see a succession of six little rooms with glass walls, each containing four cots or beds. It was smaller, cosier and a lot less scary. I smiled at the sight of little heads bobbing up and down through the glass walls but I did not spy the infamous Sister Nivern.

Three rooms down I noticed a girl in a pink nurse's uniform. She was helping a little boy with his leg in traction set up a game of dominos with another little boy who had his left arm in a cast. She looked up and saw me, and I smiled with relief. She raised her right hand and pointed her index finger and mouthed 'one minute' and quickly helped the boys start their game before hurrying down the corridor to me.

'Hello, are you the new trainee?' she called, straightening her skirt and fixing her cap back into place on her wavy blonde hair.

'Yes, I'm Sarah Hill.'

'Good to meet you, Hill. I'm Maggie Appleton. You are lucky, you've just missed doing the breakfasts, but there's plenty to do in the kitchen if you wouldn't mind helping me?'

'Show me the way,' I replied, glad to have something to do.

'Come on, the kitchen's the door at the top of the corridor. We call it the milk kitchen as it's where we make up the babies' bottles and do all the sterilising. That's the next job on the list; we'll go and give the little ones their bottles and a cuddle – nicest bit of the morning.'

I followed her eagerly as we made our way briskly towards the milk kitchen. Appleton pointed at various doors along the corridor as we passed by, telling me, 'That's the sluice, that's the linen cupboard, there are several bathrooms along here for the children, but visitors have to go to the lavatories in the hall. We're terribly short staffed today. Staff Nurse Lennard has gone to assist in an emergency case. I'll make you a cup of tea and quickly fill you in and then you can get cracking. You'll need to know the names, conditions and treatment of all the children by tomorrow when you see Sister Nivern. You're in luck; all the sisters are in a big meeting with Matron today over something or other – they don't tell the likes of us nursery nurses.'

'You're a nursery nurse?'

'Yes, we're a new-fangled idea. Sister will tell you. Nursery nurses are nothing but untrained girls paid to play with children,' Appleton said in clipped impressionistic tones and then laughed. 'Your arrival has caused a bit of a to-do already, Hill.'

'Oh, why?' I asked, worried again.

'There was a cadet nurse called Francis here until this morning, but as we've got you now, Matron's moved her on to Geriatrics. She wasn't best pleased. She's a nice girl; I dare say she won't hold it against you.'

Oh, now I was worried. I hadn't meant to push anyone out. Appleton opened the door to the milk kitchen. There was a well-rounded woman with her back to us, standing at the large sink, her sleeves rolled, elbow deep in suds. I heard the clink and slosh of the washing up as she stacked the bottles, teats and lids expertly on the draining board; the foam glistened in tiny bubbles on her shiny wet black forearm. Without deviating from her task the woman turned her head and smiled a big, whole-hearted grin.

'Oh, you perfect angel, you've done all the bottles already,' said Appleton, genuinely thrilled. 'Hill, this is Pearl, our ward maid. What she doesn't know about Infants Ward isn't worth knowing,' continued Appleton, giving Pearl a little nudge.

Pearl hooted at the compliment. 'Nice to meet you, child. I've made you girls some good hot coffee with lots of milk and sugar. You have a little break while I finish these off and then I'll be out your way.'

Appleton handed me one of the white coffee cups from the side. I sipped the camp coffee made up from concentrated liquid and boiling water; it was very sweet but it tasted good.

'That hits the spot, thank you,' I said to Pearl. She beamed back, one hand holding a dish cloth and the other resting for a moment on her large round hip as she drank me in. Her eyes were wide and dark brown and she had deep dimples in her cheeks to match her broad, beautiful smile. Though fairly short, Pearl's hair refused be constrained in a bun and thick black curls at her forehead and at the nape of her neck resisted hairpins.

'Pearl's coffee is a house speciality – get it while it's hot,' said Appleton as she took a big swig from her cup. 'It's the last one you'll get before lunch. You can go at 1.30 pm but make sure you're back for 4.30 pm on the dot, and have your tea before you come as you won't get a supper break till seven o'clock. Then you'll finish at nine o'clock if you're lucky, but you can't go until Staff or Sister say you can, and just pray they don't ask you to accompany some little darling to The London or Bart's or you won't see your bed till past midnight. Then you'll need to be back tomorrow morning at eight o'clock, bright eyed and bushy tailed. Got it?'

'Got it,' I nodded and grinned. I was doing my best to contain my excitement. Appleton and Pearl were so nice, it was such a relief. Everything was going to be fine; this was going to be great. I certainly wouldn't be back in South Wales in two weeks' time.

'I know it's a long day but most of the time if you are on at eight o'clock you are usually done by six o'clock. It's just we're very short staffed, and who'd dare say no to Sister? Not me that's for sure,' chuckled Appleton. 'What about you, Pearl?'

'Sister Nivern doesn't take any prisoners, but you be a good girl and do what she says, you'll be just fine,' reassured Pearl.

'Now Hill, shall I show you how to make up a baby's bottle or will I be teaching my grandmother to suck humbugs?'

'I have made up bottles, but it was a long time ago,' I explained. 'Please, would you show me. I wouldn't want to get it wrong.'

'No problem,' said Appleton with a grin. 'Hand me those two plastic jugs in the steriliser.' I obediently opened the door and got a face full of steam. I reached in to grab the jugs but quickly drew my hand back out: they were still far too hot. 'Sorry,' said Appleton. 'Use these.' She handed me a pair of plastic tongs. 'They cool down fast once they're out. Now all the equipment has to be thoroughly washed, rinsed and sterilised every single time,' she continued. 'Get that big tin of baby milk and get six bottles out of the steriliser and line them up.' I handed her the baby milk and she popped the lid off as I fetched the empty narrow-necked glass bottles. 'Now you measure one scoop of baby milk to one ounce of boiled water and mix it together in the jug. Never make up more than thirty-six ounces as it's too risky,' said Appleton, scooping out powder into her own jug.

'Pearl, pass Hill the feed chart so she can see how much each baby has, would you, please.'

Pearl, who had just finished the washing up and was busy getting the next load into the steriliser, handed me a clipboard showing the names and cot numbers of the babies on the ward and how much their current feed was. I noted Sister Nivern's exalted signature on the bottom of the chart; it was a spidery hand, all sharp edges and wobbly strokes. I carefully made up the feed following Appleton's instructions to the letter, under the watchful eye of Pearl. I poured the babies' milk into the glass bottles and popped on the small rubber teats which fitted snugly over the top. All done and I hadn't spilt the milk or broken a bottle.

'Now, you just pop them in the sink and cool them down rapidly before putting the bottles in the fridge,' said Appleton as she checked the amount of milk in each of my bottles against the instructions on the feed chart. 'Well done, Hill. Perfect first time,' she said, putting the clipboard back in its place. I beamed with pride.

'I'll take bays one, two, three, four and five as there's only a baby in each of them. You do six – they're all babies in there but at least you can get it done in one go. Start with the youngest, they'll need it the most,' Appleton said, lining up her bottles on a tray. 'Here, take the feed chart. It'll help you remember who has what, and learn their names and cot numbers.'

I took the four bottles Appleton had left and made my way to bay six. Four little cots were lined up, two of which were occupied by large standing infants who started to howl and thrust their arms forward on seeing me arrive with the milk. They almost snatched the bottles out of my hands and started glugging away before I could even lift them out of the cot. The other two babies were much smaller, not newborn but not far off. One was still sleeping but the other started to kick her blankets off and open and close her pink little rosebud mouth excitedly when she saw me.

I softly lifted the baby out of the cot and placed her over my shoulder, feeling her warm curly-haired head nestled in between my neck and cheek as she folded into me. I moved to the chair in the corner of the room and cradled her in my arms, putting the teat of the bottle to her lips. She started sucking wildly straight away, her big brown eyes widening as she looked contentedly up at me, her tiny black fingers wrapping themselves around my hand as she glugged her milk down. She was so beautiful, I could feel my heart pounding to the rhythm of her feed. When she finished her milk I rubbed her back in small circles as she gurgled and wriggled and did a loud unapologetic burp before falling asleep. I didn't want to put her down, she was so warm and small and perfect, but the other baby needed his feed too.

I tucked baby Mary back into her cot and checked on the older babies, who were just finishing their bigger bottles. One left me in no doubt that he was done as he hurled his empty bottle over the side of the cot and I caught it just in time or it would have smashed on the floor. The cheeky toddler clapped his hands in delight and he and his little friend started to stamp their feet and babble to each other over the railings of their cots. I tiptoed over to the fourth cot but baby Barnaby was still sleeping. I didn't want to rudely wake him up by just picking him up, so I pulled back the blanket and let the cool air do its work. I tickled his toes as he began to stir and cooed over him. I suddenly sensed someone was watching me; I looked back over my shoulder and saw Pearl standing in the doorway of the room. 'You have a good way with babies, Hill. They like you,' she said.

'I'm just making it up,' I replied, as I lifted the baby out of the cot and returned to my chair to give him a bottle.

'That's what all mothers do, child,' she told me. 'I love to have a cuddle with the babies. It warms my heart. I'll just get these washed and sterilised. You enjoy him,' said Pearl as she gathered up the empty bottles.

'I will,' I said lifting my eyes briefly from baby Barnaby's face. He was older than Mary, but his tummy didn't pop out in the same way, his eyes were a little dewy and he had dry little patches all over his skin. This baby took down his milk steadily in shallower glugs. It took much longer to give him his bottle but as he finished he went very red in the face and started to hold his breath. My heart started to quicken and my breath shorten. Oh no, what's wrong, what's wrong? I asked myself, my mind racing as to what I should do. Suddenly he stopped, tightly shut his eyes and screwed up his little face. He starting pressing his legs so hard against my stomach I thought he was going to jump out of my arms. He then passed a very loud, very hard stool and relaxed. I laughed. 'Time to change your nappy then!'

After I'd changed Barnaby and washed and sterilised the bottles, I was just thinking I'd go and see if Appleton needed a hand when the door banged open. A tall thin nurse with mousy brown hair and watery grey eyes stood in the kitchen doorway. I knew by the colour of her dress that this was Staff Nurse, just as she knew I was the new trainee nurse by the colour of mine. She didn't bother with introductions.

'Nurse Hill, follow me. We've an emergency transfer from Maternity. Get a cot ready for a new baby and then get yourself over to Maternity quick as you can. I'll be waiting for you.' Staff Nurse Lennard turned on her heel, headed off back down the ward corridor and disappeared through the doors. I could see Appleton watching her through the glass of bay five so I popped my head round the door.

'Staff Nurse says I need to get a cot ready for an emergency case from Maternity.'

'Oh right. You can make them up a cot in here. Just fetch some blankets, sheets, a gown and some nappies and plastic pants from the laundry room. Then you'll need to pick up the registration forms for Staff to fill in. There are folders and blank forms in the little cupboard to the left in Sister's office,' Appleton instructed.

'Thanks, Appleton,' I said and hurried off to get it all ready. I practically ran to the Maternity Ward. I didn't want to keep Staff Nurse waiting; and the baby – if it was an emergency transfer, the poor little of thing must be quite poorly.

I could see Staff Nurse talking with the Maternity Ward Sister in hushed tones over the little desk in the centre of the ward. I handed her over the buff folder with the blank registration forms inside.

'Follow me,' Staff said, walking towards one of the screened-off beds. As her hand reached up to pull back the green curtain she told me in a curt whisper, 'Don't say anything.'

A woman in a pink nightdress was lying in the bed on her side, her face turned away from us. Next to the bed sat a man in a brown suit, his eyes cast down to the floor. He was holding her hand; they were both motionless like in a picture. Neither of them looked at us as we entered. On the side of the bed nearest to us was a new baby, lying sound asleep in a little cot.

Staff Nurse cleared her throat. 'Mr and Mrs Williams, we are going to take the baby to Infants Ward now, if that's what you still want?' They didn't reply. Staff Nurse waited a moment. 'I have the forms here which we need to complete before I do the transfer and you will need to sign them.'

'All right,' said Mr Williams. 'Just take it, will you.'

I made a little involuntary intake of breath at the spikiness of his voice. Staff Nurse glared at me, and I looked away and tried to wipe the look of shock off my face.

'Do you want to say goodbye to her?' asked Staff Nurse softly. I saw the woman's shoulders shudder slightly but she did not turn to face us.

'We've said our goodbyes,' said the man. His voice was tight and low.

'Very well, if you should change your minds and want to see her or check on how she is doing …' began Staff Nurse.

'We won't,' interrupted Mr Williams with undeniable finality.

'Nurse, take the baby to Infants Ward,' said Staff Nurse evenly. 'I need to finish off the paperwork with Mr and Mrs Williams.'

I picked up the sleeping baby and wrapped the blanket round her tiny body and began to cradle her as she stirred and then relaxed in my arms, continuing her slumber completely unaware that she would never see her parents again. I looked at her mother's back and willed her to turn around and look at her baby. I wanted Mrs Williams to snatch her child back from my arms and hold her close, but she didn't. She didn't say goodbye, she didn't look, she didn't move a muscle.

I hurried away from the bed, from Maternity Ward and Staff Nurse and Mr and Mrs Williams, holding the slumbering infant her own father had referred to as 'it'. She hardly weighed a thing; she was so light in my arms, so helpless and small. Tears pricked at my eyes and I held my breath until we were back in the safety and familiarity of Infants Ward. I now allowed myself to look into her face. Something was not right with this poor baby. Her heavy eyelids were tightly closed, and I could see the rise and fall of her tiny chest as raspy breaths came out of her thin mouth. I cuddled her to me and closed my eyes, my chest contracting and heaving with suppressed sobs.

Appleton was waiting in bay five playing a game of peepo with the toddlers. I crept in to join her, sad to break up their happy game.

'Who have we here?' she asked gently.

'A little girl. I don't think she has name. Her parents are called Williams.'

'Well, let's get her settled. It'll be visiting time soon. Her mummy and daddy will want to see she's well taken care of.'

'I don't think they will, Appleton,' I whispered. Appleton arched an eyebrow and took a closer look at the baby. 'I mean, I don't think they want her. I think they've abandoned her.'

'Let's wait and see what the doctor says. Maybe they'll come round. Here, give her to me,' said Appleton, taking the little girl and rocking her in her arms. 'Why don't you go to the linen cupboard and fetch baby an extra blanket.'

I quickly made my way to the large linen cupboard off the ward corridor. I switched on the light and saw shelves and shelves of neatly folded white linen stretching out in front of me. I shut the door very firmly behind me and ran my hands over the piles of blankets until I found the softest one. I could still feel the warm spot on my chest where I'd held that little baby so tightly to me. I picked up the blanket and hugged it and wept. I hadn't been in Hackney for twenty-four hours but I knew that the way I saw people and life had changed forever. Bless Appleton for knowing I needed to be alone for just a moment. There was such goodness here, but there was more sadness than I had ever imagined, and it wasn't even lunchtime yet.

3

I left the hospital with heavy steps as I trudged back to the nurses' home in the dark. What a day! What had I let myself in for? I wanted to curl up in my bed and brood over the day's events, but as soon as I set a foot in the lobby I met Wade practising her shuffle-ball changes on the polished wooden floors. She took one look at my drooping head and ordered: 'Upstairs and get changed right now. You're coming with me to the pub.'

Before I knew it I was slinking down the back of the hard wooden bench in a booth tucked away in a darkened corner of the Adam & Eve public house. The gloomy saloon was lit by heavily fringed, dusky pink hanging lamps, and grubby red curtains were drawn at every window and doorway. Just visible in between the curtains, empty bottles, half-full glasses and a throng of Hackney locals was a dull patterned wallpaper, curling at the edges. My eyes lazily traced the tree-pattern around the room from the main entrance to the vacant stage.

Later I'd come to love the Adam & Eve, how the hospital staff drawn from all corners of the Commonwealth stood back to back with the barrow boys from the markets with their greased-back hair and familiar patter. That rock and roll and Elvis battled via the juke box against the songs of the West Indian sailors from the docks who came to meet their nurse girlfriends. That union men from the factories shouted politics and talk of strike and equality in between pinching the bums of the two blonde barmaids. And how the burly landlord, Alf, kept mugs for regulars hanging up over the bar so they could enjoy their pint in their favourite tankard and take comfort that this was their local, their East End, a little piece of security in a rapidly changing world.

But right now I just felt the weight of the day pressing down on me. I kept wondering how that poor little baby was doing on Infants Ward. Was she hungry, or crying or sleeping? Did her nappy need changing? Who was holding her, singing to her and giving her all the love that she was missing out on? I'd stayed with her for the rest of my shift. I didn't go for my breaks; I just couldn't leave her – she'd already been abandoned once that day. Pearl had brought me toast and tea to keep me going as I sat through my fruitless vigil – I kept hoping Mrs Williams would come rushing through the door and reclaim her baby, but she didn't.

When it was time for my shift to finish, I was in the middle of giving the baby her bottle. Staff Nurse came and scolded me. 'Nurse Hill, you can't just give all your attention to one child. We have eleven children right now that also need care. What about them?'

'Yes, Staff Nurse Lennard.'

'Your shift's finished now. You can go. Be back here on the dot of eight tomorrow morning.'

'I'll just finish giving her this bottle,' I'd replied.

'If you must,' huffed Staff as she bustled off.

I didn't care that it was time to go. The baby fed so slowly and I wanted to make sure she got the opportunity to get as much as she needed. I didn't care how long it took. When she finally finished I winded her gently, rubbing her back as she softly snored into my ear. I sat holding her tight for about twenty minutes, just rocking ever so slightly from side to side until she went into a deep slumber, and then I tucked her back into her cot. The poor little thing didn't even have a name.

I was jostled out of my reverie with a nudge from the nurse at my side, Fiona Lynch. She pointed to Wade, who was laughing up at the bar.

'She's been there so long she'll have forgotten what you're having,' Lynch chided with a smile playing on her lips.

'I don't mind,' I said quietly.

Wade had deposited me with Lynch, who was having a quiet drink with another student nurse. I saw them roll their eyes as Wade approached, but Wade either didn't notice she was butting in or she didn't care as she launched into her short to-the-point introductions.

'Hill, this is Lynch and Maddox. We're all on the same corridor so I'm sure you'll be the best of friends,' said Wade. 'Shove up, girls, Hill's had a hard first day on the job and needs a drink. What'll you have, pet?'

'Ginger beer,' I said meekly as I wished for a vodka and lime, but I was only seventeen and didn't want to get Wade into trouble.

Wade snorted. 'Ah bless your heart, a ginger beer then,' she laughed as she sauntered off to the bar to order herself a brandy and Babycham.

Lynch smiled at me and shuffled up to make room on the bench next to her. She had bobbed brown hair with a full fringe and light brown eyes. I was to find she was a little like me, with a knowing smile, always ready to tease and make us all laugh. Maddox lifted her mousy brown head briefly from some pamphlet she was reading as she chewed a long strand of hair in her mouth. She maintained a slightly neglected look, matched by the holes in her green jumper and long-legged jeans. She gave me a brief tight smile and returned to her reading.

'First day, is it?' asked Lynch.

'Yes.'

'Bit of a tough one, was it?'

'Not all of it. Some of it was unsettling. It's just, I didn't know, I've never seen …' I couldn't get my words out.

'You soon learn fast. I think you see the worst and the best of people in a hospital. I'm still getting used to it myself.'

'You're new too?'

'I started in the summer along with Maddox here. What ward are you on?'

'Infants Ward.'

'Ah, you see – best and the worst. I'm one of seven, so long before I started nursing I already knew my way round a bottle and a nappy, but the stuff you see! The suffering some people go through, you can't help but be a little shocked. What sort of person would you be if you weren't?'

I found the soft tones of Lynch's lilting Irish accent immensely comforting as she continued to commiserate with me. 'What you need to remember, Hill, is that we nurses are there to give care and comfort. Everyone needs a bit of that, and they'll not get it from the doctors. You are on that ward for a reason, to give all the comfort you can to those children because, let's face it, you won't know one end of a thermometer from the other yet. It's such a shame some of those poor little mites do not have the love of their mothers and fathers, but you can't change that.'

Maddox lifted her long down-turned nose out of the pamphlet she had been engrossed in. She pushed her round black thick-rimmed NHS spectacles back into place on her nose as she nodded in agreement. 'Lynch is right. You cannot let it get to you, or you will never get any work done and then what use would you be to the patients? It's their pain, not yours. You cannot go crying in the linen cupboard every five minutes.'

'How did you …' I muttered.

'We all need to shed a few tears from time to time,' Lynch added quickly. 'I've excused myself for a little weep in the cupboard many a time; it's the only place you can get any privacy. God, we're only human.'

'What I'm saying is,' continued Maddox, undeterred from her theme, 'if you want to change things you have to look at the bigger issues. Why do parents walk away from their children? Why are landlords allowed to let out houses you wouldn't keep a dog in? Why are women and immigrants treated as less important than white men? It is all part of the same problem,' preached Maddox as her index finger tapped away on her leaflet.

Thankfully Wade finally rejoined us with the drinks. 'Here you go, Hill. Sorry it took so long; I was waiting for the slow barman to find out if they had any ginger beer.'

After a few drinks, a bit of chat and a lot of laughter things started to feel much better, and that warm feeling of belonging I'd had with Appleton and Pearl in the kitchen returned. There was a group of housemen at the bar. Wade was flirting with them as she went up for drink after drink. I kept to my corner, chuckling with Lynch and not understanding half of what Maddox preached, sticking to the ginger beer. Wade eventually sauntered back with a houseman on each arm. 'This is Freddy and Guy. Doctors, may I introduce Lynch, Maddox and our newest addition fresh from the Sorbonne, Hill,' slurred Wade. 'Sit yourselves down now, lads; come on girls, make some room,' she instructed as Freddy sat on my left and Guy on Lynch's right, squeezing us together in the booth.

'So, were you at the Sorbonne?' said Freddy with a tone of condescension, pushing his wavy brown hair out of his insipid blue eyes.

'Wade's joking,' I replied. I saw his eyebrow arch as he heard my Home Counties Good Girl boarding school accent. Not what he had been expecting. 'My cousin's there though,' I muttered under my breath as I took a sip of my drink.

'Right,' he said, sitting up straighter and moving the hand that had been grazing my thigh on to the table to take up his pint glass. 'What ward have they put you on?'

'Infants Ward.'

'I'm starting Infants Ward as part of my rotation next week. I'll be there till Christmas.' I didn't say anything. 'You'll have to keep me on the straight and narrow, Sarah,' he whispered.

'Deviate from the right side of things often, do you?' I said.

'No, no. I'm a good chap, you know. Play the church organ, organise concerts to raise money for sick children, that sort of thing.'

I half smiled at him but I didn't catch his eye. I was already finding this Freddy a bit tiresome. If I'd wanted to be fondled by a public school fop I could have picked up one of my big brother's friends. 'Why don't you let me show you what a nice chap I am? Let me take you out on your day off.'

'I don't know when that is.'

'I can wait. Chances are, if I'm nice to Sister Nivern, I might be able to swing us having the same day off.'

'We'll see,' I replied, but already my attention was being drawn away by the sight of Wade drifting over to a group gathered by the juke box as the intro of 'Ob-La-Di Ob-La-Da' blasted out. I took in the horrified faces of Lynch and Maddox as Wade hoisted up her skirt and nimbly ascended from a chair to the top of a small round table in the centre of the saloon bar. The intimate crowd clapped her on as she kicked up her legs, showing her stocking tops, and sang along with John, Paul, George and Ringo.

'She carries a tune well,' said Freddy, very amused.

'Oh my God, she's at it again,' said Lynch, cringing and covering her face as we watched Wade tap dancing and doing high kicks as she hopped from table top to table top.

'Time to go,' Maddox instructed calmly, taking off her glasses and putting them and her pile of literature into a square black handbag.

'We can't just leave her!' I protested, but they were already making their way to the door.

'She'll be fine,' Lynch assured me, putting her hand gently on my arm. 'She's a regular turn. Wade thinks she's still on at the Empire when she's had a few.' I couldn't wipe the look of surprise and amusement off my face as we made our way through Wade's overly appreciative Hackney audience and scuttled out of the pub back to the nurses' home, happily losing Freddy and Guy in the crush as they held back to enjoy the show.

4

A knot was tugging in my stomach as I nervously fidgeted on a chair in Sister Nivern's office the next morning, watching her slowly pour out two cups of tea from a white pot into pale-blue china cups and saucers.

'Sugar?' she asked.

'No, thank you,' I replied in a small voice.

'Good. Nasty habit to take sugar. I think it smacks of weakness,' she said with a thin-lipped smile as she passed me my cup. My hand shook just a little as I took it from her and sat it down in front of me on her desk. I watched Sister Nivern take a long sip of the hot tea.

'Ah, that's better,' she sighed. 'I do like to start the morning with a good strong cup of tea. None of this coffee muck. Nasty habit taking coffee in the mornings – I blame the American GIs bringing it with them during the war. Among other things,' she added, this last sentence more to herself than to me.

'Hmm,' I muttered into my tea as I took a tiny sip. What a strange, strange woman, I thought. She reminded me of Sister Cecile from the Convent. She too was overly tall, thin and bony. All sharp elbows, a jutting jaw and a pointy chin. I had deplored the way the nun had cosied up to the rich and famous parents on Prize Giving Day; I never liked Sister Cecile, though she clearly was keen to impress my father.

'I've been looking through your file, Nurse Hill,' continued Sister Nivern. 'I must say I'm surprised you applied here. A girl with your education and background should be at The London or Bart's at least. You've got eight O-levels, girl.'

'I wanted to be where I could do the most good, Sister,' I said firmly.

'Well, that's all very commendable, Nurse. But take it from me, women like us never really fit into a place like this.' I didn't say anything. I just wanted to drink my tea as quickly as possible and get out.

'Staff Nurse Lennard tells me you looked after our newest patient most diligently yesterday. I've assigned you to bay four today. It does not pay to get too attached to any particular patient, do you understand?'

'Yes, Sister.' My heart lurched at the thought of not spending my shift with Baby Williams, but I grudgingly admitted to myself that she had a point.

'I want you to ensure everything is shipshape in your bay before Drs Manning and Warren, our paediatricians, make their morning rounds at nine o'clock. Then there will be Mr Duncan, our orthopaedic surgeon, on his rounds at ten o'clock.'

'Yes, Sister.'

'Staff Nurse Lennard will be observing you. You'll find her waiting for you in bay four.'

'Yes, Sister.'

I bobbed slightly and exited Sister Nivern's office and went without delay to bay four as instructed. I was glad I'd already checked on Baby Williams before reporting to Sister at 8 o'clock on the dot. I could see through the glass there were only two little boys in the bay. One was eating his breakfast at a small table with great gusto, despite having his arm in a cast, and spraying crumbs everywhere. The other child, a toddler, was standing up in his cot drinking a large bottle of milk. All this was taking place in relative silence (if you ignored the slurping) under the watchful eye of Staff Nurse Lennard. I smiled at the boys as I breezed in and tried to look like I knew what I was doing.

'Good morning,' I said.

'TPRs first, Nurse,' barked Staff.

Before I could stop myself I asked, 'TPRs?'

Staff said with exasperation, 'Temperature, Pulse, Respiration.'

Note to self: don't show your ignorance, Sarah. I wouldn't make that mistake again. I walked up to the empty bed nearest the door and looked for the boy's chart – I could not find it. Staff Nurse Lennard watched me fruit-lessly search for the chart for a minute before she informed me curtly, 'Medical charts are locked in Sister's office; we don't want to lose half our records by having them ingested by a toddler, do we?'

She explained sternly, 'What you need is the day's observation sheet. Ensure it is written up and added to the main
records by the end of your shift and that the next day's top
chart is prepared and in place for each child. Make sure it is
updated thoroughly throughout the day or we won't know
where we are tomorrow, will we?'

'Yes, Staff.'

'Begin,' she instructed as she stood by the wall. I noticed
she did not lean on it, but stood rigid and straight,
maintaining an inch between her frame and the wall at all
times. No one could accuse Staff Nurse Lennard of taking
the weight off.

'Good morning, Sam,' I said cheerfully to my first patient.

'Hello, Nurse,' he said through a mouthful of cereal,
spraying milk all over the table.

'Do you need any help?' I asked. I thought I heard Staff
faintly tut, but I wasn't certain.

'Nah,' he replied as he paused from eating and then took
a large gulp from his beaker of milk.

I returned to reading his notes. His diagnosis was '#green-
stick. Result of falling off slide in Victoria Park.' What was
a #greenstick when it was at home? I would ask Lynch when
I got back to the nurses' home; something to do with his
broken arm, surely. I was not going to give Staff the satisfaction of showing my ignorance again.

'How's your arm today?'

'All right,' he chirped.

'Are you going to start the observations, Nurse Hill?'

I looked at the blank spaces on the sheet and then glanced surreptitiously into the other bay through the glass to where another nurse was doing her morning observations. She was holding a child's wrist and looking at her watch. I'd taken the odd pulse at the children's home in Wiltshire during my Voluntary Service when the children were unwell. I could do this; I just had to remember how to record it.

'Hold out your hand, please, Sam,' I instructed my little patient. He huffed slightly. I took his small hand in mine and felt for the pulse just under his thumb and felt it beating. I looked at my little upside-down nurse's watch and counted the beats for 30 seconds.

'Pulse 52, Staff,' I reported. The miserable besom didn't respond in the slightest.

I flipped over the top sheet and looked at the previous day's record; it said *100 bpm*. Why had his heart rate dropped so suddenly? Was that bad or good? Think logically, Sarah, I scolded myself for panicking. All right, *bpm* was beats per minute. I'd counted for only 30 seconds … why did I do that? I thought, and tried to remember six months back when I'd been shown how to take a pulse: because you just double it. So 52 times 2 was 104 bpm. I took the blue pen from my top pocket and scribbled it down with an air of satisfaction, '104 bpm, so that's all good. Now your respiration; just breathe in and out for me, that's right.' I stood by his side watching the rise and fall of his chest and checked he wasn't holding his breath to count his respiration and jotted that down too. Just his temperature to go.

I glanced around the room searching for the location of the necessary instrument. In the far corner was a small glass case hanging on a bracket with three thermometers inside it, each in a thermometer-shaped glass case of its own. I went over and took the one with Sam's name on it, pulled it out and instinctively gave it a shake as I walked back. I wasn't sure why I was doing this, but I was fairly certain it was what you did, something to do with heating up the mercury perhaps.

'And why do you suppose we keep the thermometers there?' asked Staff Nurse Lennard.

'To keep them out of the reach of little inquisitive hands, Staff,' I replied. Again, she said nothing. I had to take heart that I must be doing all right so far; I didn't doubt for a second that if I did anything even slightly wrong she would immediately put me in my place.

'Arm up now, please, Sam,' I instructed as I slipped the thermometer in his armpit and kept him steady with my hand on his shoulder to keep it in place. Then I looked at my watch. 'Now, keep as still as you can for a minute and a half, please, Sam.'

I watched the little hand tick around the small face of my nurse's watch. '98.4. Your temperature's just fine.'

I scribbled *milk, toast, scrambled eggs and cereal* in the section for fluids and food on his chart. I'd done it. First task of the day done – one more to go. I was just about to put his notes back when Staff Nurse Lennard sprang into action and took them from me. She looked over my notes.

'Good work, Nurse Hill. I'll leave you to carry on with observations. After that you need to ensure they are washed, dressed and have taken their vitamins and medicine before doctors' rounds in half an hour. Chop, chop.'

'Yes, Staff,' I said as confidently as I could as she strode off to monitor the morning checks in the other bays.

'Snap,' shouted Sam as his Queen of Spades went down fast on my Queen of Hearts. It was just after lunch and we'd been playing on and off since the morning rounds. Sam and I sat on either side of his bed, while little Cecil – who was in with a poorly tummy after drinking disinfectant – was having his afternoon nap.

'You've won all my cards,' I laughed as he piled up the deck as his winnings.

'Can we play again?'

I looked at my watch. 'Well, it will be visiting time in fifteen minutes. We'd better check you've got all your things ready. Doctor said you could go home today, remember?'

'Oh, do I have to?'

'I'm afraid so. Come on,' I said as we went to see what he had in his cupboard.

Staff Nurse Lennard appeared at the door. 'Is that child ready to be discharged?'

'Almost, Staff,' I replied.

'Good. You're needed in bay three. Nurse Patel needs a break.'

I obediently followed her to bay three. Two older babies were in cots covered in large cotton tents. There was a constant billowing of mist and vapour from two steam kettles in the corner of their tents. An Indian nurse I recognised from the nurses' home was refilling one of the large copper kettles. It spat and hissed at her. She looked rather fed up.

'Patel, you can go for your break now,' instructed Staff Nurse Lennard.

Silently Patel hurried away, wiping her hot face and pushing her frizzy hair off her brow and neck where it was clinging onto her skin.

'You'll need to do their TPRs before visiting time in ten minutes,' instructed Staff. 'The steam makes them make quite a fuss but I wouldn't let Sister Nivern catch you cooing over them if I were you,' she said before disappearing almost literally in a puff of smoke.

The two babies were whimpering. It must have been horrible in all that steam. I picked up their notes to see what called for all this. Georgie Edwards and Bobbie Fry were nine and ten months old. They had both been diagnosed with bronchitis. I guessed the steam was to try and clear their little chests.

It was so hot under those cotton sheets. Both boys were fractious – overheated and bothered by the steam and the noise from the hissing kettle, and finding it difficult to breathe with a constant involuntary cough as they tried to clear their chests. It must have been so frightening for them, in their isolation, away from their mothers, in this strange place.

Two women, their arms linked, hovered in the doorway.

'Can we come in, Nurse?' asked the taller of the two.

'Yes, are you relatives?'

'Georgie's mine, and Bobbie's hers,' she replied.

She took a few steps forward but the other mother remained in the doorway.

'I can't today, Kathleen. I just can't,' she cried and then hastened off back down the corridor.

'She'll be all right once she's had a fag. It'll steady her nerves,' said Mrs Edwards as she pulled back the cotton tent and lifted out her baby. 'Would you give little Bobbie a cuddle so he don't feel left out?' she asked.

Together we sat in the chairs and patted the children dry with towels, trying to soothe them.

'It's very hard when all they do is cry. Lizzy, my sister, thinks he doesn't love her any more,' Mrs Edwards explained. 'And she thinks it's her fault, our fault that the babies are sick.'

'Why do you think the babies are sick?'

'It's our house. Our landlord won't fix it. The walls are mouldy, the floorboards are rotting. We all of us cough our guts up every night.'

'Have you nowhere else to go?'

'Both our ma and pa are dead. My husband's never out of the pub and hers walked out on her while she was in labour with Bobbie here. I've got my factory job back, but someone has to stay home with the boys, and that's her. I just don't make enough to get us somewhere better.'

'I'm sorry.'

'Not as sorry as I am, Nurse. This is the second time they've been in with bronchitis and I don't expect it to be the last,' she sighed.

I didn't know what else to say. Could the house really be so bad? Would the council let a house like that stay standing, let alone house a family with small children? No wonder Bobbie's mother felt wretched and helpless. How was it right that those children were forced to live in a home that made them ill? Surely there must be something I could do to help, but I didn't know what.

Visiting time was almost over and back on bay four there was still no sign of Mrs Briggs to collect Sam. I was keeping him amused with a game of I-Spy when Staff Nurse Lennard bustled in.

'Mrs Briggs made an appearance yet?' she asked in such a way it insinuated that Sam's mother's lack of maternal concern was my fault.

'No, Staff Nurse Lennard,' I replied feebly.

'Well, I suppose I'd better telephone her myself then,' barked Staff.

'Not on the phone,' chirped Sam.

'Did I ask you, Samuel?'

'Nah.'

'Then please keep your opinions to yourself.'

'Nurse Hill, if Mrs Briggs isn't here by tea time we shall have to call the constabulary and ask them to call on her.'

'She won't answer the door to a peeler,' said Sam.

'That's quite enough from you, Samuel, thank you,' scolded Staff.

'She always makes us hide under the bed when a copper comes a-knocking, or the rent man, or my dad,' said Sam.

I wasn't getting a very favourable impression of Mrs Briggs from her offspring. He was only four going on fourteen by the sounds of it. Then I heard the clip-clop of heels echoing down the corridor, and my eyes widened as they drank in the sight of a woman with a huge platinum blonde beehive tottering towards us at a half gallop. She wore very high black boots, a fluffy white coat and clutched her shiny black handbag to her chest.

'Please don't tell me, I've missed visiting hours again,' she cried breathlessly as her hands stretched out to either side of the doorframe of the bay for support. 'I've barely seen hide or hair of my boy since he came in. These visiting hours are a killer.'

'Just in the nick of time, Mrs Briggs,' said Staff coolly. 'Samuel is ready for you to take home now.'

'He can't come with me now. I'm not ready. I thought he'd be in at least a week,' she said as she bent over holding her side and trying to regain her breath.

'Well, luckily for him Doctor says it's a very clean break and is mending nicely.'

'Can't you keep him till tomorrow? Only I've made a date with a chap to see *Carry On Again Doctor* at the flicks tonight.'

'Suits me,' said Sam. 'What's for tea?'

'See, he wants to stay,' said Mrs Briggs, ruffling her son's mop of golden curls.

'That is hardly the point,' Staff informed her tartly. 'His papers are ready for him to be discharged. If you would follow me to Sister Nivern's office now, please.'

Glumly Mrs Briggs trailed out in front of her, taking heavy sulky steps. 'Come on, Sam, we're not wanted,' she called to her child.

'Oh well,' said Sam as he picked up his little bag and coat with his one good arm and followed his mother.

Cecil was still slumbering; no one had been to visit him either. I popped my head into bay three where Mrs Fry had rallied and joined her sister, and Patel was back *in situ*.

'Would anyone like a cup of tea?' I asked.

'Please, dear. Both milk with two sugars,' replied Mrs Edwards.

'Righto,' I said, overly cheerful as I scurried off to the milk kitchen. I could see Doctor Warren was in with Baby Williams as I walked past the last bay. I looked back. Cecil was still out for the count; I had a bit of time. I went into the milk kitchen and got Cecil a bottle of cow's milk and made Mrs Edwards and Mrs Fry their tea. Sister Nivern was on a break so I figured there was no harm in letting the parents have a little longer with their babies. I kept the door half open so I wouldn't miss my chance with Doctor. As he was leaving the bay I came out of the milk kitchen and almost bumped into him.

'Steady there, Student Nurse, steady. You'll have me in Casualty,' he said with a smile as he made a bit of a show of checking himself over.

'Sorry, Doctor.'

'No harm done,' he said as he finished patting himself down.

'How's Baby Williams?'

'Who?'

'The baby girl in bay five, doctor.'

'Hmm, oh, the hydrocephalus with spina bifida, there's not much hope there I'm afraid, but still we persevere.'

'Hudrpceha … spina …' What was that? I couldn't even say it.

'How long have you been here?'

'It's my second day; I don't start PTS till January.'

'Your ignorance is excused then. Water on the brain with deformation of the spine.'

'That's why her parents don't want her?'

'I wouldn't know about that. But I suggest you use the nurses' reading room tonight to read up on it, rather than seeing your boyfriend,' he condescended as he swept off down the corridor with a slight swish of his white coat.

Appleton popped her head out of the next bay.

'He fancies himself a bit, doesn't he?' I said.

'Don't they all,' she said, rolling her eyes.

I tutted and popped the tea round to bay three before hastening back to bay four. Little Cecil was just getting to his feet and calling out for his bottle.

After supper I followed Dr Warren's lofty advice and made use of the medical books in the reading room of the nurses' home. I was trying to understand just what was so wrong with baby Williams that her parents had given her up. It was not a comfort to uncover what was in store for my charge; it left me cold the way those matter-of-fact books foretold of 'increasing pressure inside the skull resulting in progressive enlargement of the head, convulsion, tunnel vision and mental retardation'. I imagined the look of horror on Mr and Mrs Williams's faces when the doctors revealed their child has been born with an open spinal column. Had they refused to hold her immediately or had it been later when the enormity of their baby's condition had sunk in? I remembered their stillness, their inability to look at her – she was already dead to them. It was too horrible. That poor baby, why was she born to suffer? I firmly closed the book and put it back on the shelf and made my way back up to my room.

Later, when I emerged from the bathroom in my nightie and dressing gown, my sponge bag in hand ready for bed, I was surprised to find Maddox on all fours inspecting the skirting board outside my bedroom. Wade was hopping from foot to foot shouting in a high-pitched voice at Maddox as she was shuffling along down the corridor on her hands and knees.

'Whatever is the matter with you, girl? Bringing a rodent into the house and you want to be a nurse. You should be a keeper at the zoo,' wailed Wade.

'Stop being hysterical, Wade,' said Maddox in a calm voice without looking up at her accuser.

'What on earth is going on?' I asked.

'Maddox has lost her hamster,' Lynch said with a wry smile.

'Oh. I took hamsters to school. We found one in the head girl's water jug once after it had been missing for three days,' I told them.

'Oh my God, what's that?' cried Wade as she started stamping her foot.

Lynch picked up the now flattened object. 'It's the wrapper from a chocolate with a bit of fluff stuck on it,' she informed them softly, shaking her head.

'I wouldn't be surprised if you had rats, the state your room is in, Maddox. The cleaners can't even get in to vacuum the floor it's so covered in old tights, magazines and sweet wrappers. Cleanliness is next to godliness and that goes double for nurses,' chastised Wade.

'Found him!' shouted Maddox, triumphantly reappearing holding a golden fluffy ball of fur. Everyone piled into my room for a closer look.

'He's very cute. Can I hold him?' I asked.

'Of course,' she said.

'Make sure you wash your hands very thoroughly afterwards,' said Wade, peering over Maddox's shoulder.

'What's his name?' I asked.

'Dilly.'

'Dilly. Oh, we always called our hamsters Hamish,' I said.

'As in Dilly Dosser,' she said.

'After those hopeless hippies?' said Wade, her loathing of
both the hamster and the hippies increasing further by their
now close association.

'I was being ironic, actually,' corrected Maddox.

'The squatters that were evicted from that big house in
Piccadilly at the weekend?' I asked. I was impressed. I'd seen
it on the news. My parents had been less than approving of
these drop-outs who were living in London's empty
mansions. Better than living in squalid little houses that give
your children bronchitis, or having no home at all, I thought.

'Maddox has been seeing a young busker called Gerald
who was squatting in that office building on Russell Square,'
chipped in Lynch.

'Maddox, you dark horse!' My opinion of her was
improving.

'Yes, but now thanks to the fuzz he's homeless,' sulked
Maddox.

'I think it's terrible how they've been treated. Like they're
evil. They called them hell-raisers on the news. Well, I think
I saw a little bit of hell today on Infants Ward. Needing a
decent home to stop your babies from dying, that's hell. I
don't see what harm the hippies are doing. They don't want

to hurt anyone – they just want to change things that need changing.'

'Exactly, Hill. No harm at all. But the police, the news, the government, they are all in it together to make them the villains. Whereas it's really the establishment who are the real villains.'

'Where is Gerald now?' I asked.

'He's taking his meals at the soup kitchen run by St Barnabas over the road.'

'Gosh. So he is really homeless?'

'Yes, of course. That's the point, isn't it – to show smug people in their little semi-detached homes with tidy lawns and a tarmac drive how many people don't have a home at all.'

I thought about how I'd helped my dad put the gravel down on our drive one weekend over the summer. I felt a bit guilty at the thought of Gerald and all the others who had been thrown out. It wasn't fair.

'Did you see the report from Shelter earlier this month? Over three million people in this country are in need of rehousing due to poor living conditions. People need decent homes at a fair price,' Maddox informed me.

'There are two little boys on Infants Ward in those cotton steam tents because their homes are damp,' I told them.

'And you can bet your life they'll be discharged and sent back to the same place that made them ill and they'll be back on the ward by Christmas. It'll never end unless we demand decent homes for everybody,' Maddox explained.

'Yes, I see what you mean.'

'Well, if you're really interested, Hill, you should come with me to St Barnabas one evening and meet Gerald.'

'Maddox, have you gone mad?' Wade scolded. 'Hill's a nicely brought up young lady. She doesn't want to be taking tea with a lot of hobos.'

'No, I'd love to, thank you, Maddox.'

'Well, watch your handbag if you do go,' advised Wade. 'Early start in the morning. I'm going to my bed.'

'Night, Wade,' we all chimed.

'I better put Dilly to bed too,' said Maddox, taking the small hamster off me as she followed Wade out of my room. I went to my tiny sink and squeezed some toothpaste on to my toothbrush and started to get ready for bed.

Lynch leaned on my bedroom door, her fingers lightly drumming on the wood, I could see her reflection in the glass. She was looking at me quizzically.

'What is it?' I asked with a mouth full of foamy paste.

'Are you really interested in what some hippy has to say about homelessness, or is that just good manners?'

I thought as I swilled my mouth with water and spat out into the sink. 'I really am interested,' I told her reflection in the glass. 'The patients you see, this is their home, their world. I need to understand it better if I'm to really help them.'

'You should have been at The London.'

'Don't say that. I really want to be here, Lynch. I really do. It's not second best to me. It's so exciting. I think I've felt more alive in these last two days than I have my whole life.'

'Give it two weeks.'

'That's what my mother said. But she's wrong,' I said with a smile.

'They'll make a nurse of you yet, Sarah Hill,' Lynch whispered as her hand turned the door handle.

'I do hope so,' I giggled. 'Sweet dreams,' I told her as I pulled back the covers and fell into bed. I was asleep within minutes.

5

I soon settled into the routine of Infants Ward. We watched children come and go and come back again and tried to do our best for them. Some of the nurses were amazingly compassionate and caring, but there was a harshness to hospital life too. Many nurses and doctors did the physical care but had no time for cuddles, or kindness or fun. It was already late October and I was learning the ways of the ward and more importantly the sometimes strange ways of Sister Nivern or, as we had started to call her of late, Sister Skinflint.

Appleton and I were giving diluted welfare orange juice to the toddlers when little Flo knocked over her cup, making a huge puddle on the floor. 'Never mind,' said Appleton as she went to get some paper towels to clean up the spill.

'Never mind, never mind,' repeated two-year-old Flo.

'What do you think you are doing?' The spindly frame of Sister Nivern was in the doorway to the bay, her eyes burning into Appleton as she mopped up the juice from the floor.

'Cleaning up Flo's orange juice, Sister,' answered Appleton in a matter-of-fact way.

'I can see that,' barked Sister. 'First of all, why are you giving infants juice when I have told you water will suffice, and second of all, why are you using paper towels when you know it is so expensive? Have I, or have I not, told you before to use the cloth mop from the laundry room? That's ten shillings worth of paper you've used already. At this rate you'll be singly responsible for bankrupting the NHS.'

'Yes, Sister,' said Appleton, rising to fetch a disgustingly germy but cheap and reusable mop from the laundry room.

'And as for you, Nurse Hill, I would have thought a girl with eight O-levels would know better.'

I gave Appleton a sideways sympathetic smile as she departed to fetch the mop, only to be followed by Sister Skinflint who lectured her all the way down the corridor. I pulled little Flo onto my lap and rubbed Vaseline into the beautiful little plaits that covered her perfectly round head. She had the biggest brown eyes and though she was only just two years old we had a lovely game of catch. I thought to myself this child is going to be a natural athlete as she passed the ball back and forth to me without dropping it from the other side of the bay.

'Now, what do I have to do to get you come and watch me pass a rugby ball?' interrupted a man's overly confident voice. I looked behind me and there was Freddy, the young house-man from the pub. He'd been pestering me for a date but I wasn't keen. I had noticed Lynch in the café window with his friend, Dr Guy Fleming, only the previous week, but Lynch hadn't said anything so I'd kept that little piece of gossip to myself. I couldn't be bothered with Freddy and flirting right now so I ignored him and carried on with my work.

'Forgotten me already?' he asked, a hint of real disappointment in his plummy tone.

'I'm very busy, Doctor …' I didn't know his surname. Oh, heck. Had he told me his full name?

'MacDonald, Nurse Hill,' he said formally before slumping against the wall in self-pity. 'Do you remember my name, even?'

'Yes, it's Freddy,' I replied in exasperation.

'Well, that's something I suppose,' he said, brushing an invisible speck from his white coat and standing up straight. 'Now, what about that date you promised me?'

'I didn't promise you anything,' I told him sharply without looking at him.

'I beg to differ,' he said, edging closer towards me.

'You can beg all you like,' I retorted, popping Flo back into her cot and then loading the children's breakfast things onto a tray with a bit of a thump. I swept past him out of the bay and to the kitchen. As I started to fill the sink up with water he appeared again. For heaven's sake!

'You wash, I'll dry,' he told me, taking up a tea towel from the draining board. He was trying to be charming and helpful, like a hero in a film – it wasn't working.

'Surely a doctor has better things to do with his time,' I said, taking the tea towel from him as I set about vigorously washing up with a clatter, attempting to drown out the sound of his drivelling chat-up lines. But before he could give me another facetious answer the door opened and Sister Nivern entered the kitchen.

'Nurse Hill, stop wasting Dr MacDonald's time,' she scolded. Freddy sauntered up to her full of self-importance and smiled, pushing his wavy hair off his forehead. Sister blushed slightly as he towered above her. 'I'm sorry, Doctor,' she apologised sycophantically as she did to all the doctors.

'That's quite all right,' said Freddy the weasel, enjoying the effect his public school boy looks were evidently having on her. 'I was just asking Nurse Hill if she had noticed any change in the little black baby's condition.'

He didn't even know their names. He hadn't even looked at Flo. What sort of doctor was he?

'Nurse, there's plenty of laundry that needs doing at once. Appleton's already in there and don't dilly-dally chatting,' snapped Sister. Clearly I was no longer needed for this sickening *tête-à-tête*.

'Yes, Sister,' I said, annoyed, yet relieved to be away from Dr Freddy MacDonald. If he thought I'd go on a date with him after that little performance he'd got another think coming.

I found Appleton in the laundry room already ironing the newly washed clothes. I went to the mending pile and picked up a needle and thread and started to sew.

'Why can't these go to the hospital laundry and save us the extra work?' I asked as I attempted to thread the cotton through the eye of the needle.

'Sister Skinflint thinks they'll ruin them and then she'll have to buy new and there'll be more expense,' said Appleton, pressing the iron down hard with each piece of information. 'It's one thing to give us extra work, but the children could do with a little orange juice every day just for the vitamin C and she wants them to have nothing but Adam's Ale.'

'Talking of ale, fancy a brew?' I asked.

'Water's just boiling,' she said, relaxing a little. 'Would you pour, dear?'

'Of course, dear,' I giggled as I moved the heavy laundry baskets to one side to reveal a box full of cups and saucers, a packet of tea, a teapot and a little jug of milk. I helped myself to some freshly boiled water and poured us both a much-needed cuppa.

Appleton and I each took a big sip as we sat on an old crate enjoying a breather. 'Ah, that's better,' sighed Appleton. 'I was gasping. What did you get exiled for?'

'Talking to doctors, I think. Though to be honest I was glad to be away. An impudent houseman after a date, if you please,' I replied. 'We could do with getting a stash of biscuits too,' I suggested, trying to change the subject.

'Is he good looking?' asked Appleton, never one to be easily deterred.

'In a public school foppish sort of way, if you like that sort of thing,' I said petulantly as I pictured Freddy's smug face and the revolting way he'd cosied up to Sister Nivern.

'Do you like that sort of thing, Hill?' asked Appleton rather directly.

I thought. 'Not really, no.'

Appleton was just about to ask me another question when we heard footsteps approaching.

'Quick, hide the tea things,' instructed Appleton, springing up and back to the ironing board. I just managed to hide everything behind the baskets and take up my mending once more when the door opened to reveal Sister Nivern.

'Nurse Hill, those bronchitis boys were discharged this morning and the mothers forgot to take their medicine. I want you to take their antibiotics and give clear instructions on the dose. It's one of those should-be-condemned slums on the other side of Victoria Park. Appleton, go with Hill. You'll be safer in a pair,' instructed Sister, giving us a paper bag and the address scribbled on a little piece of paper.

As we stood in front of the one-up one-down tumbledown house rented by Mrs Edwards and Mrs Fry I couldn't help but shiver despite my cloak. The doorsteps along the street were littered with either broken bottles or wrappers, and children wailed inside battered old prams outside their peeling front doors, next to overflowing rubbish bins. Grubby-looking washing fluttered in the wind on clothes lines strung up from the windows. There were no trees, not a shred of green space, not even a yard. Dirty water from broken guttering ran down the walls of the crumbling houses and tiles were visibly missing from the roofs all along the row.

'No wonder those children are sick,' I whispered to Appleton.

'I know. Imagine the agony of bringing your baby back here knowing it'll make them sick again.'

'What sort of landlord rents a place like this?'

'One who knows he'll get away with it. Cost of housing keeps going up and it forces the people who can't afford it into these slums.'

We knocked on the door. I could hear the familiar crying and coughing of little Bobbie and Georgie. I didn't know what was worse, keeping them safe but away from their mothers in hospital or sending them home to this. Mrs Fry answered the door with Bobbie in her arms. He was red faced and pummelling his mother with his fists.

'What do you want?' she shouted over his screaming and wheezing.

'You forgot the boys' medicine, Mrs Fry,' I said.

'Is that a crime?' she snapped.

'They'll need to start taking it tonight. All the instructions are on the bottle. Shall I talk you through the dosage?'

Mrs Fry snatched the bottle out of my hand. 'Do you think I'm stupid?'

'No, no, of course not,' I muttered. Oh, help. Then fortunately Mrs Edwards appeared dressed in her hat and coat.

'Who's there, Lizzy?' she called to her sister.

'Those nurses from hospital come to check up on us.'

'We haven't come to check on you,' said Appleton softly. 'We just didn't want you to have the bother of coming back to the hospital for the antibiotics.'

'That's your story,' insinuated Mrs Fry as she retreated back into the dilapidated house with her distressed child.

'Don't mind our Lizzy,' Mrs Edwards consoled. 'Now I've got to get to work. Bye, Georgie, take care. Lizzy, make sure you give the boys their medicine, like the nurses told you,' she called back into the darkness of the hallway but there was no response. She sighed and shut the door behind her. We stood together on the street. 'You going back to the hospital?' she asked.

'Yes,' I replied.

'I'll walk with you as far as the park,' and we set off. I was at a loss as to what to say as I walked between Appleton and Mrs Edwards.

'Where do you work, Mrs Edwards?' asked Appleton.

'I'm in the rag trade,' she replied, and something told me not to pry any further. We walked the rest of the way in silence. I was sure there was something she wanted to tell us but I didn't know how to open up the conversation. At Victoria Park she left us, and Appleton and I waited until she was out of earshot to talk.

'Did you feel like there was something she wanted to tell us?' I asked.

'Yes. Why didn't she just come out with it?'

'I don't know; pride perhaps, or fear? It must be very hard to leave her baby, and Mrs Fry doesn't seem like she's coping with Bobbie, never mind Georgie.'

'I think she's depressed,' said Appleton.

'Who, Mrs Fry?'

'Yes.'

'If only they could have a decent place to live. Is there really nothing we can do?' I exclaimed.

'There's the Lady Almoner. She finds homes for people sometimes.'

'Like she's doing for Baby Williams?'

'Yes. She might know of some housing. There's a lot of building going on, they're forever knocking things down and digging up the road.'

'Should I ask her, do you think?'

'Sister Skinflint would have a fit. You can't go over her head.'

'OK. I'll ask Sister Skinflint,' I said, resolved. 'She must see how sick the children are. Nothing is going to make them better if they don't get a proper home.'

I had my mission. As soon as we were back at Hackney I went directly to Sister Nivern's office and knocked on the door. 'Enter,' she responded. And there she was sitting at her desk having a cosy afternoon tea with Freddy.

'I've just come back from taking the antibiotics to Georgie Edwards and Bobbie Fry's house, Sister.'

'Well, you've had a nice little day trip. Get on with your work, Nurse.'

I saw Freddy smirking into his teacup as I stood in front of them, like a girl sent to the headmistress's office.

'I've seen for myself the condition of their home, Sister. It's not a fit place to keep a dog, let alone two very sick babies.'

'I didn't realise you were training to be a housing inspector as well as a nurse, Nurse Hill.'

'If you could see if for yourself I'm sure you'd agree with …'

'See it for myself? I am not accustomed to visiting the lower orders in their slums, Nurse Hill, and neither are you. It is how they live. I dare say it is quite shocking but they are used to it.'

'But, Sister, the babies will never get better living there. If you would just speak to the Lady Almoner about whether she could find a more suitable home for them.'

'You may have eight O-levels, but I think you are a long way off from telling me what I *ought* to do.'

'Yes, Sister,' I replied, shrinking back. I'd really messed this up. I didn't care for myself, but those babies and their poor mothers – I wanted to cry.

Freddy put down his teacup and put his hand on Sister Skinflint's arm. 'I am sure it is just youthful exuberance on Nurse Hill's part, Sister. I think what she's saying is she is coming to you for your experience and because she knows the influence and high regard the Lady Almoner has for you. Isn't that right, Nurse Hill?' I nodded. 'One little word from you and I'm sure you could transform the lives of that family,' continued Freddy.

Sister Nivern lost all interest in me; her gaze was entirely fixed on Freddy. A slow smile spread across her thin face. 'I suppose I could mention it at some point to the Lady Almoner. Leave it with me, and not another word on the subject. You may go.'

'Yes, Sister,' I answered, grateful to get away.

I felt sickened at the sight of her and Freddy. Not because I was jealous, but it was just wrong somehow. I wanted to find Appleton to talk to her and figure out how I felt. Freddy had just helped me and yet I didn't feel grateful, but surely I should. Surely he had just done a kindness to Mrs Fry and Mrs Edwards? Oh, well – what did I care? It was time to get the bottles ready for the next feeds. I went into the milk kitchen and mechanically got the tin of baby milk down and started to make up the bottles, but once again Freddy sought me out.

'You'll get me into trouble again,' I snapped as he came in.

'I thought I just got you out of trouble,' he answered back smoothly.

'Thanks for that.'

'You're welcome. I'd say one good turn deserves another.'

'Oh, really.'

'Surely you can see I'm not such a bad chap. Let me prove it to you. I've got tickets to see *Forty Years On* at the Apollo Theatre. It's a cracking good show, I'm told. Have you seen it?'

'No.'

'Then you'll come?'

'When is it?'

'24 October.'

'I might not have the night off.'

'You leave that to me. I've got old Skinflint wrapped around my little finger.'

Again I couldn't think of another excuse. So I ended up saying yes to a date with Dr Freddy MacDonald, the public school, organ-playing, rugby-tackling fop. Not what I'd envisaged for my first romance in Hackney, not at all.

6

'Wade, you're blocking the telly,' Maddox shouted at Wade, who was springing about as usual in front of the big black and white television.

'I knew it, I knew it. I've put on so much weight since I started midwifery; all those boxes of chocs from grateful parents – here, don't give me any more,' she shouted, chucking a huge box of Weekend at me, the chocolates and candies scattering into my lap and onto the chintzy sofa in the nurses' sitting room.

Lynch scooped up a big handful, 'She's not saying you're fat, she's saying you're blocking our view of the telly.' She popped a toffee in her mouth. '*Monty Python's Flying Circus* will be starting in a minute and we don't want to miss it. If I wanted to see a musical-hall act I'd have gone to the Palladium.'

'More of your hippy anarchist rubbish, I suppose. I want to watch *Randall and Hopkirk* on ITV. I don't know what the BBC's thinking, giving these posh lefty lads a slot on the telly. They're traitors to their own class.'

'Where did you hear that load of old twaddle?' chimed in Maddox, probably sticking her oar in because of Wade's hippy-bashing.

'I read it in the *Radio Times*, as it happens,' said Wade primly and unconvincingly.

'Oh, then it must be true,' snorted Maddox.

'Don't you laugh at me, girl. I'm old enough to be your mother; my son's your age. You students should speak to us professional nurses with a bit more respect.'

'You may be as old as my mother, but you act like my thirteen-year-old sister at the best of times,' crowed Lynch.

'How dare you?!' screamed Wade.

'Now steady on, you two,' I interjected, my eyes flitting from Wade to Lynch, neither looking like they were going to back down. 'You're quarrelling over nothing. Wade, sit down, come on.'

'I'll not stay where I'm not wanted,' spat Wade.

But Lynch couldn't resist, saying calmly, 'It's never stopped you before.' Wade stormed out of the room shouting, 'You're nothing but a bunch of silly little girls.'

'What's got into her?' said Maddox as she got up to change the channel on the television set.

'Who cares?' said Lynch. 'She's nothing if not a drama queen. A woman her age should have a bit more self-respect.'

'I like her,' I said quietly.

'Hill, you're as soft as butter, you like everyone,' Lynch chortled.

'That's not true.'

'Oh, no. So how do you feel about Dr Freddy MacDonald then?' teased Lynch, taking a long stylised drag on her Consulate cigarette and blowing the smoke out over my head.

'Oh, yes. You went on a date with that Hooray Henry last night,' said Maddox, joining us on the sofa. I had Lynch on one side, Maddox on the other – there was no escape.

I shoved a chocolate in my mouth. 'He took me to see *Forty Years On*,' I told them, munching hard.

'Did you see John Gielgud?'

'No, it was somebody else. It was very good.'

'And how was Freddy?' said Lynch, tucking her feet up underneath her on the sofa and leaning in for every detail.

'Nice. Bit of a show-off. Tried to make out how expensive the tickets were *but I was worth it* and all that tosh.'

'But hospital staff get them for free!' Lynch told me.

'I know,' I said.

'What did he do when you told him he was a liar?' asked Maddox.

'I didn't,' I replied.

'Why not?' she said, disappointed I'd failed to unmask him.

'Because I won't get anywhere by showing him up. But now I know.'

'What do you know?' said Maddox, reaching into my lap and taking a handful of Wade's chocolates.

'That he's not entirely on the level.'

'Hill, where does that get you?'

'It gets me rid of a pest, eventually. A pest who happens to be a favourite of Sister Skinflint and could make life diffi-cult for me on Infants Ward before I've even begun my Practical Training. If I just wait, he'll show himself up, his sort always do, and then he'll be the one avoiding me, just you wait and see.'

'Sounds like a funny strategy to me. Why don't you just tell him to get lost?'

'Just not my style,' I told them. 'Now, *Monty Python*'s starting so stop with the interrogation, would you?'

After the show, which we all loved and vowed to watch every week, I wandered out of the sitting room and made my way up the big spiral staircase. I could hear music playing; it grew louder and louder as I climbed the stairs and I realised it was Freda Payne singing 'Band of Gold', the volume turned up full blast. A group of angry nurses were gathering outside my room in their nightdresses and dressing gowns, some with their hair up in rollers, others taking the opportunity to have one last smoke before bed. One angry little blonde nurse in a pink frilly nightie with cold cream all over her face was banging on Wade's door with her fist.

'If you don't turn it down right now, Edie Wade, I'll get Home Sister,' she shouted.

There was no reply.

'What's going on?' I asked an African girl who was lean-ing on my door, lighting up.

'Wade's been playing that bloody song over and over again. It's a good tune but after the fifteenth time you start to get a bit sick of it, you know what I mean,' she told me, offering me a cigarette from her pack.

'No, thank you, I don't smoke,' I said.

'Suit yourself. I find it's the only way I can relax before bedtime.'

'Shall I try and talk to her? She was a bit upset earlier.'

'Well, we guessed that.'

I edged forward and waited for the blonde girl to stop her banging.

I tapped on the door. 'Wade, it's Hill. Would you open the door, please?' There was no reply. 'I don't think she can hear me over the music,' I said. I barged through the nurses blocking entry to my room and knocked on my bedroom wall. The music continued. I tried again.

'Got any more bright ideas?' said the pushy blonde, who'd come into my room without an invitation.

I leaned out my window; it was a little more than an arm's length to Wade's bedroom window.

'Could one of you get me the pole for opening the bathroom windows, please,' I asked. A Malay girl who lived a few doors down dashed off and returned with the long pole with a hook on the end. On my chair was a headscarf Wade had lent me one night when we were coming home from the Adam & Eve and it started to rain. I tied it to the pole and stuck a note on.

Edie
If you don't stop that racket they'll throw you out the nurses'
home. Let me in and we'll talk.
   Sarah

I opened my window and started edging the pole towards Wade's room and tapped on the glass. It didn't take long. I felt her grab the pole and when I drew it back both the headscarf and the note were gone. There was a sudden screech of the needle being drawn across the record and the music stopped.

'Well, thank heaven for that,' said the frilly blonde, and one by one the girls all dispersed back to their rooms. I waited till the coast was clear before gently knocking on Wade's door, and this time she let me in.

Her room was an absolute mess. Clothes, stockings, shoes and other bits and bobs were strewn all over the floor and bed. Ripped-up papers were scattered across the desk and the chair was tipped over on its side. Wade was half undressed, her lipstick was smeared across her upper lip and chin and rivers of black mascara ran down her cheeks. She stood in the room swaying from side to side, a half-empty bottle of vodka in her hand.

'Edie, what's happened?' I gasped.

'It's Bill,' she wailed, taking a huge swig of vodka.

'Your husband?' I said. From the little Wade had told me I knew the pair had long been estranged.

'He's got some jumped-up solicitor to write to me saying he's divorcing me; didn't have the guts to tell me himself. My boy, Tommy, wrote to me. Said his dad's taken up with some hippy chick half his age. Got her in the family way and he's going to marry her,' she blurted out. 'Tommy says there's no place for him at home now, and I don't have a bed to offer him, so he's only gone and signed himself up for the Royal bloody Navy,' she wailed. 'What have I done? Why did I come to London? I've lost everything. I've no home, no husband, no son, nothing.' Wade broke off in huge great big sobs, sinking onto the single bed. I walked to the little sink, washed out a tumbler, filled it with water and sat down next to her.

'Here, drink this,' I said gently, passing her the glass.

She took small breathy sips. After a long silence she said thoughtfully, 'Bill was such fun when we first met. Mam never liked him, and we fought like cat and dog, but I did my best. I always tried to make him happy, but he chased every bit of skirt that came his way. Didn't matter how hard I tried, he was always staying out all night and spending my housekeeping on other women and drink.'

'Sounds like you're better off without him,' I said.

'Am I though? I'm past forty, I know I don't look it but I am. I don't want to come home to an empty bed night after night. A woman needs a bit of comfort, she needs to feel appreciated, she needs to feel loved, or what happens to you? You become like Home Sister, some old drunken biddy alone in a room with no one to care for you.'

'You've still got Tommy,' I sympathised, feeling increasingly uncomfortable and out of my depth with this topic of conversation.

'Have I heck. He'll be off round the world; I'll be lucky if I see him once a year for the next ten years. And then he'll find a nice lass, and what woman wants her mother-in-law about?'

'Why don't you write to Tommy and ask him to visit before he sails?' I suggested.

'Do you think he'd come?' she asked, looking up at me, a glimmer of hope in her eyes.

'I'm sure he would.'

'He's not got two brass farthings to rub together,' she whimpered, rubbing her eyes with an old handkerchief she'd found on the bed. Suddenly she sprang up and went to look at her face in the mirror and started to wipe the make-up off with a damp cloth. 'Of course, Tommy will have to sleep on the floor,' she plotted.

'Oh, Wade … I don't know …' I babbled, before she fixed me with those big china doll eyes.

'You wouldn't tell on me, would you, pet?'

'No, of course not,' I said, completely outmanoeuvred.

'You'll just love him, he's only a year or two older than you,' she chirruped.

Feeling a touch careworn but glad I'd prevented Wade being turned out from the nurses' home once and for all, I got up to go back to my own bed. As my hand reached for the door handle, I said, 'Wade, you're really better off without Bill. He sounds like an absolute bounder. You can do much better than him.'

'Oh, do you really think so, at my age?'

'Of course. You're an attractive woman. You've literally got a spring in your step.'

'You're right. I'm not letting Bill Wade get the better of me. I've a day off tomorrow, I'll take myself down the West End and get myself a new fella.'

My eyes widened but I didn't say anything. That woman's certainly got bounce, I thought, as I wearily returned next door to my own room.

7

A few nights later, as Maddox and I made our way down the steps of the nurses' home into the frosty night air, she tugged my coat sleeve and pulled me to one side.

'Look, there's someone lurking in the bushes,' she whispered.

I clapped my gloved hands together and stamped up and down impatiently, trying to keep warm, and peered half-heartedly into the gloom.

'Maddox, you're imaging things. It's Bonfire Night so if you are trying to give me a fright for Halloween you're a few days too late,' I said, pulling her with me down the path. I was in no mood for silly games as my second date with Freddy loomed ahead of me.

Already there were a few whizzes and bangs overhead as eager children from the neighbourhood let off the odd early firework. As we crunched our way down the gravel path in the direction of St Barnabas, a lone rocket lit up a dark corner of the lawn for just a moment and I too saw there was indeed a shadowy figure by the bushes, half hidden from view. I peered closer, trying to make out who it was, but I could only see the glow of a cigarette tip.

'Do you think it's another Peeping Tom?' I whispered to Maddox.

'Well, if he is he's not going to scare me,' she said, suddenly filled with gusto at the thought of a snooper getting an eyeful of our fellow nurses. She stomped off in the direction of the unknown lurker, now dragging me behind her. 'We see you, come out now!' shouted Maddox when we were about fifty yards away. 'We've already called the police so there's no escape,' she lied.

'What did you go and do that for?' shouted back an alarmed but familiar voice, and I gave a huge sigh of relief as Wade stepped into the light.

'What the devil are you doing there, Wade?' barked Maddox rather harshly.

'Mind your own beeswax,' Wade snapped back. 'What are you doing sneaking up on people? You gave me a terrible fright,' she said, all the time keeping her eyes on the side gate.

'We gave *you* a fright,' shouted Maddox. 'What silly games are you playing now?'

'We thought you were a prowler but we haven't called the police,' I explained.

Wade made a little tut, but she wasn't engaging. Though I could see she was bristling all over, she wasn't up for a stand-up row with Maddox tonight, and that in itself was out of character for Wade, never mind the lurking in the bushes on a freezing cold November evening. 'Well, you can see it's just me having a quick fag, so you Nosey Parkers can be on your way now, can't you,' she said, dismissing us, all irritated and distracted.

This wasn't like Wade. What was she up to? 'Is everything all right?' I asked. I was evidently not very skilled in the art of interrogation yet, as of course the answer was, 'I'm fine,' and then she clammed up and turned away from us completely. So, now not scared but feeling rather curious, Maddox and I continued on our short journey over the road to the church.

'Do you believe Wade was just having a cigarette?' I asked Maddox.

'Not one bit,' she snorted.

'What was she up to?'

'Probably meeting up with some fella and trying to sneak him into her room. It wouldn't be the first time. She's been out on the town every chance she gets lately.'

'Yes,' I said, thinking back to the previous week. Appleton had got tickets to see Tom Jones at the Hammersmith Palais and Wade had tagged along. Appleton just loved the Voice from the Valleys and had stared in horror as Wade scrambled up onto the stage during 'She's a Lady' and handed him a pair of French knickers. She'd tried to plant a kiss on his knee before she was dragged off by a rather hefty-looking bouncer. An hour later it was chucking-out time and Appleton and I had searched for the unruly Pupil Midwife everywhere, ducking our heads under toilet cubicles doors and venturing into dark sticky corners full of dodgy men groping inebriated girls all in the name of the Free Love. Eventually we'd given up and went to retrieve our coats, only to find Wade snogging the bouncer in the cloakroom. Edie had taken no heed of our entreaties to come away with us, and in the end Appleton told me, 'She's a grown woman. Come on, let's go back to mine. It's too late for you to get the bus back to Hackney on your own.'

So we'd made our way together, giggling and recounting the concert and Wade's escapades, until we'd reached her little house in Stoke Newington. It was nearly one o'clock in the morning and her dad was waiting up for us. When we'd walked in a little tipsy and full of high spirits he didn't scold us; instead, he'd given us a big grin and said, 'Good night, girls? I'll make you some beans on toast.'

A little crowd was already gathering in the church at St Barnabas for the concert and fireworks party. Freddy was in the doorway handing out programmes, dressed in a smart suit and tie, his hair freshly cut and his shoes shining with extra polish. Standing directly opposite Freddy was the shambolic figure of Gerald, Maddox's boyfriend. His long curly brown hair was desperately in need of a wash. There were holes in his green woollen jumper and he still had his brown Mac on. His shoes were all scuffed at the toe and his thick black-rimmed glasses were held together at the joints with sticky tape. I liked Gerald. I enjoyed our chats in the Adam & Eve and had eventually discovered why he was opting out of the private housing market – his own father was a big property developer and landowner and he'd always felt sorry for his family's tenants. He wanted to stand as an MP and do something to change the world.

I could see Gerald was getting on Freddy's nerves already. 'No one's come to hear your left-wing manifesto,' I heard Freddy snap. He'd have been all over Gerald if he'd known his father owned half of Derbyshire. 'People have come to hear music and enjoy a party, not to listen to your claptrap. Go and sit down now with the rest of the tramps,' Freddy told him, and then he saw me. 'Ah, Sarah, come and sit with me at the organ; I need someone to turn my pages. You don't want to be in the cheap seats with the rest of the riff-raff.' He took me firmly by the elbow and dragged me off towards a shadowy corner of the choir stalls.

I looked back in anguish at Maddox but she was already getting stuck in with an undeterred Gerald, the two of them in matching green jumpers and faded jeans, handing out leaflets and asking people if they had an indoor loo. I felt overexposed in my black and white mini dress and wished I was in the old pair of white jeans my younger sister's boyfriend had given me when he'd got too podgy for them. I knew Freddy was looking at my legs and I didn't like it.

'Scoot down,' Freddy instructed me, pinning me between the stone wall to my right and behind me, the organ in front of me, and Freddy himself to my left – there was no escape.

Freddy flexed his large pale fingers in front of him, pressing them together and cracking his overly big knuckles. He dramatically pressed down on the keys and his legs started working the pedals. His thigh was pressing into mine and he felt indecently close, especially in a church. I started to feel all hot and flustered and the music was washing over me. It was so loud there, virtually on top of the organ. Then I realised what he was playing. 'Freddy, that's Procol Harum, isn't it?'

'"A Whiter Shade of Pale", yes it is.'

'Pop music in a church?'

'It's sacred music, based on Bach, and let's not forget the vestal virgins in the lyrics and all that,' Freddy said, turning his face to look at me, a twinkle in his eye. I stared straight ahead. 'Page please,' he instructed me and I obeyed. He twiddled a few knobs on the organ and turned to me without a hint of irony and said, 'If music be the food of love …' Oh God, was this him pulling out all the stops? This was going to be a long concert.

I was getting hotter and hotter, and then suddenly I couldn't breathe and the 'Hill tickle' struck – I started coughing uncontrollably. People started to stare. I was competing with Freddy's music and he didn't like that. He twisted slightly to let me squeeze past. My miniskirted bottom was practically in his face, but I didn't want to think about that, I just wanted to get out. I ran down the aisle feeling a hundred judgemental eyes on me, and out of the big church doors into the welcome embrace of the cool night air. I took long deep breaths and eventually the coughing subsided. I heard the music from the concert echoing off the stone walls of the church but I didn't want to go back inside just yet. Instead, I wandered round the edges of the churchyard looking at the gravestones, reading the names and dates on each tomb just like we did as children on a Sunday morning after church.

Hovering by the wall of the churchyard, I noticed the side gate to the hospital grounds was open and a man was being let in. I swear it was Wade who was giving him the come hither. So Maddox was right, she *was* sneaking a man into the nurses' home! Oh well, I thought, her and half the corridor. Even though men were forbidden I hardly ever made my way up to the fourth floor without passing some chap or other. But for all her talk of Free Love and Women's Lib I hadn't noticed Maddox inviting the homeless Gerald back to her room for a nightcap, so maybe she was just envious of Wade. Sometimes I wished I could be as carefree as Wade was.

I joined Maddox and Gerald for the party in the Church Hall but I decided not to mention seeing Wade with her mystery man. They were already deep in conversation with the vicar – well, they were talking and the vicar was nodding along. Freddy came over to join us, bringing me a glass of warmish cider from the refreshment table just as Gerald was in full flow.

'I'm not saying Harold Wilson couldn't be doing more, of course he could,' said Gerald. 'There are so many scandals. But at least Labour has put a stop to leaseholders losing their homes without compensation with the Enfranchisement Act. People round here are still paying what amounts to a small fortune to slum landlords for properties I wouldn't keep a pig in. We need the state to build decent homes for people at rents the ordinary man can afford.'

'And woman,' chimed in Maddox. Quite right, I thought, taking a large slurp of cider; it was mainly women after all who had to fight the tide of illness that resulted from poor housing – look at poor Mrs Edwards. How many babies did we have on Infants Ward right now who wouldn't have been there at all if they had a nice home with proper sanitation and heating? How was that asking too much?

'And women,' Gerald corrected himself. 'You tell me how can we do what is needed fast enough when every time we legislate the Tories oppose. They always have and always will defend the power and privileges of the few and to hell with working men and women and their children. Tell me, Vicar, didn't Jesus tell us to look after the poor, to treat those less fortunate than ourselves we respect?'

'Yes, he did,' began the vicar, but Freddy interrupted.

'Now, now, you can't go using Jesus to support your watery argument,' he said. I finished my cider and picked up another cup, looking for pain relief from this awful so-called date. 'Jesus didn't know London would be flooded with people fresh off the boat day by day. And all right, maybe some of these places round here aren't exactly the Ritz, but think of where they've come from. I bet an English slum is a damn sight better than an Irish slum, an Indian slum or a West Indian slum. I bet to *them* it is the bloody Ritz.'

I felt my blood boil. 'As a nurse I see it as my duty to be ready to meet the needs of all my patients regardless of *who* they are. Isn't it the same for doctors?' I asked Dr Freddy MacDonald.

'Yes, but we aren't talking about hospital, we are talking about government, Sarah. Keep up.'

'Doesn't government have the same duty of care for everyone within our borders just as in the hospital walls?'

'Well, that's a bit of a simplistic view,' dismissed Freddy.

Maddox told him, 'Hill's right. If things were more equal our society could afford to meet the needs of all its members. Society should not discriminate against minorities on grounds of religion or race or colour. There should be decent housing for everyone; slums and overcrowding must be dealt with; immigrant ghettoes must not be allowed to develop. There should be work for those who seek it, not just in London but right across the country.'

'Well that's a very nice little dream,' said Freddy patronisingly. 'But not everybody wants it; whereas every man wants a bit more cash in his pocket, and that's the way I vote. It's the way any man with sense and a grip on reality votes. I want to hang on to what I've got and see it grow. I'm not risking the likes of Harold Wilson giving away what's mine to some layabout.'

'You'll be eighteen soon, Sarah,' said Gerald. 'You'll be able to vote in the next general election. You still undecided?'

I had already made my mind up I was going to vote Labour, but before I could say so Freddy told me, 'Vote the same way your old man does. Best thing any girl can do.'

Uncomfortable with the turn our conversation had taken, the vicar tried to defuse the tension and said, 'I do believe the fireworks will be starting soon. Please, help yourselves to sausages and buns. I just need to check how the bonfire is doing. Excuse me.'

We all helped ourselves to a few sausages and a few more cups of cider, and the tension of the political debate began to subside. I could feel the warming effect of the alcohol and started to feel a little mellower. Freddy and some of the other housemen were singing to keep the crowd amused, and you couldn't deny it, he had a very good voice. I started to drift gently from side to side as he sang 'A Whiter Shade of Pale' again, his eyes burning into mine with intensity and meaning. I heard the first bang of the fireworks and we all rushed outside in excitement to watch them light up the night sky. They were so pretty and I felt cheered and light. Freddy took off his jacket and placed it round my shoulders to keep me warm and I felt his arms coming round my waist to keep me steady. I felt heavy and a little woozy, and all the words and the music jumbled round my head so I couldn't think straight any more. I let myself lean my weight on to him just for a moment to try and collect my thoughts once more. I drank in the spinning of the Catherine wheel, round and round in a burst of glowing flames that shot off in all directions. Freddy held my hand and led me into a quiet

Sarah Beeson

corner to enjoy the view as a fresh symphony of fireworks, whizzes and bangs started again. I could smell his freshly washed hair and the touch of his hand circling mine and then before I knew what was happening Freddy kissed me.

'Then what happened?' asked Appleton as she loaded up the steriliser in the milk kitchen.

'The fireworks finished. I pulled away from Freddy; I felt like I was going to be sick.'

'Sick from the cider or sick from the kiss?'

'Both,' I said, looking at my shoes. 'I just felt so angry. Angry with him and angry with myself,' I huffed.

'Then what happened?' she asked, slamming the steriliser shut.

'I stomped off through the muddy graveyard and went home.'

'Did he come after you?' said Appleton, as she handed me a much-needed cup of coffee.

'No, thank God. When I was a safe enough distance from him I glanced back. He was just standing there with a smug look on his face.'

'What will you say when you see him?'

'As little as possible,' I replied, before taking a satisfying slurp. 'I'm just going to give him the cold shoulder for a bit.'

'Do you think that'll work?' Appleton asked, leaning on the counter opposite and lifting her soft blue eyes to mine questioningly.

'No, but it's all I can come up with right now.'

Appleton sighed and looked concerned. 'You look tired.'

'I just lay in bed last night, running over and over it in my head. Was it my fault? Was he really that bad? Had I given him the impression that I liked him by wearing that mini-dress? I wish I'd worn an old pair of jeans. I didn't think.'

'It was just a kiss; don't beat yourself up about it.'

'A kiss from a man I actively despise! I've really let myself down.'

I don't know why but my dad's face popped into my head. He wouldn't have cared about the cider – growing up in various parts of the countryside we were always having some sort of local brew, but how had I ended up feeling like bloody Freddy MacDonald was my boyfriend? A doctor: wouldn't everyone be thrilled? I could get married now and give up this nursing malarkey. Wasn't that why girls went into nursing, to try and bag themselves a well-born doctor so they could put their little feet up in a nice house in the Home Counties? Well, not me. Not me.

'And now he will think I like him. Or does he know how I feel and thought he'd try his luck anyway?'

'From my experience of doctors they think we're all swooning over them, regardless of the reality of the situation,' advised Appleton.

'I am never going on a date with a doctor again, ever.'

'Did you get any sleep?'

'Well, I was just drifting off when I heard a tap-tapping at my door. It was Wade. She wanted me to help her sneak out the chap she'd brought into the nurses' home last night. Be her look-out and check the coast was clear. Only it wasn't some old sea dog like I thought, it was a young chap sleeping on her floor. Turns out it was her son, Tommy.'

Appleton started to laugh. 'Well, that's a relief, I suppose.'

'It is a bit.' I smiled for the first time that morning. 'I need to get two tablets for my headache; can you cover while I pop to the nurses' cloakroom?'

'Bit of a hangover?'

I nodded and went in search of a little pain relief. It was going to be one of those days, I could just feel it.

I was having a sit down on the hard wooden bench of the nurses' cloakroom waiting for the paracetamol to work its magic when I heard a 'Brumm, brumm, beep, beep,' coming out from behind the stack of coats and cloaks. I bent down and saw a pair of scuffed knees and a line of little cars on the floor. I drew back the mountain of cloaks to see a mass of red curls and four-year-old little Annie Donnelly turned her freckled face up to see me with a broad grin.

'Hello, Annie. What are you doing in here?' I asked.

'Getting some peace and quiet,' she answered primly.

'I see.'

She scuttled out from under the coats on her hands and knees, pushing a row of toy cars and vans in a procession along the floor with her one good arm; the other was in a sling.

'Nee nah, nee nah, nee nah,' she sang, running her toy ambulance up my knee. 'Look, my dad bought me a

Doolance,' she told me proudly. Her dad was a mechanic; they shared a love of cars. 'I came in a Doolance when I hurt my arm. The boys wanted to have it, but it's mine. They don't have a Doolance but they can't have mine,' she told me firmly.

'Is that why you're in here?' I asked her. She nodded. 'Do you want to help me give the babies their bottles? I could do with a helper today.'

'Please,' she answered, squeezing my hand and laying her head in my lap, her beaming face turned up towards me.

'Come on then,' I said, taking her by the hand. 'Shall I keep your Doolance safe in my pocket?' She nodded again and gave me her precious toy ambulance.

The last baby on the feed chart was Baby Williams. Annie came with me into the bay and played with her ambulance, cars and vans quietly on the floor – she'd had enough of passing me the bottles and cooing at the babies. Baby Williams must have looked strange to her; she wasn't like a little doll to play mother to as the other babies were. I too was experiencing a growing sense of despair at the change in Baby Williams's appearance. Over the past few weeks her head had increased in size and the pressure of the fluid on her brain meant she was getting less and less responsive; her eyelids were drooping and she barely made a sound any more. The problems with her spine meant she had a stillness that even for a baby put people on edge. I gently lifted her out of the cot and went to sit in the chair where we'd shared our first cuddle on my very first day all those weeks ago. I held her little hand and spoke to her, and whereas before her eyes had followed me and she'd perked up, today there was nothing.

Today was our last day. The Lady Almoner, the hospital social worker, had found her a place in a home – where she would be clothed, fed and watered until the inevitable happened, which the doctors had said wouldn't be long. She didn't finish the bottle; she fell asleep again and I couldn't rouse her to take just a little more of her feed. I put her back in her cot and looked around for what else I could do for her before she left us. Nothing; there wasn't even anything to pack. This child didn't have a gown or a bottle to call her own. I led Annie away from this room, it was too sad. I closed the door on Baby Williams. I would never see her again; it turned out that she didn't live to see her first Christmas.

Suddenly Freddy, Wade and the night before seemed terribly unimportant. It was so unfair that a little baby could suffer so much and the rest of the world just carried on – even me. I promised myself that to me every baby I ever met would be precious and important, no matter what the circumstances. It was easy to love the fortunate babies, the healthy ones with nice mums and dads, but who was there to love ones like Baby Williams? To the Lady Almoner or Sister she was just another bit of business – not a person. I wanted every child to matter, to be loved; to me, that was what would make the world a better place.

8

Sister Skinflint was only working a half day, and with her out of the way we'd let some of the parents stay on a little longer. I was with Annie and her dad doing a tea round when Freddy turned up.

'Knock, knock. Nurse Hill, could I have a word with you for a moment?' said Freddy.

'I'm busy right now, Doctor,' I replied coolly.

'That's all right. You go, we're fine,' said Mr Donnelly.

'I haven't finished the tea round,' I explained.

'I'll do that for you, love,' he kindly offered.

I searched for another excuse but Freddy stepped aside for me to leave the bay. 'If you'd come this way please, Nurse,' he instructed and I glumly followed.

He indicated we should step into the linen cupboard but there was no way I was going with him in there. Instead I made for Sister Nivern's unoccupied office with its large glass window making the occupants safely visible to the whole of Infants Ward. Freddy shut the door behind him but he didn't step towards me; instead he rested on the inside of the door, blocking my exit and keeping himself hidden from prying eyes.

'Alone at last,' he said, raising his eyes hopefully to meet mine.

I quickly looked away. 'How can I help you, Doctor?'

'Very formal,' he grunted.

'I'm on duty,' I scolded.

'So am I,' he said petulantly, like one of the children.

'Freddy …' I started but I didn't know what to say.

'Don't you like me any more?' he asked.

I don't know if I've ever liked you, I screamed inside, but I didn't say anything. I just let my eyes search for help through the window, hoping to see Appleton, hoping she'd come and rescue me.

Suddenly the doors at the end of the ward flew open and in came three men, one with a half-naked child in his arms – the bottom half – with a cross-looking nurse from Casualty running after them. I knew the nurse. Her name was Kaur; she was even shorter than me and she had a temper on her. You wouldn't want to mess with Kaur, but even she looked flustered. The phone rang and I answered it.

'Infants Ward,' I said, picking up the receiver.

'This is Casualty. There are three men coming up with an eighteen-month-old boy,' Casualty Sister told me.

'Yes, they've just burst onto the ward corridor,' I told her.

'For heaven's sake. Where's Kaur?' she barked.

'She's with them, but there are three of them and one of her, and big strapping chaps they are too.'

'Who is this?' asked Sister.

'Hill, Sister.'

'Listen here, Nurse Hill. That poor little boy has burnt his bottom very badly on an electric fire. He's very distressed. Those men insisted on bringing him up after the doctor had seen him on Casualty only minutes ago; wouldn't even wait for a porter or papers or anything. When they arrived in Casualty they in fact marched up to the first man they saw in a white coat and insisted he see the child immediately or they'd punch his teeth out. It was a radiologist. They had the poor man up against the wall before I pointed out to them that he wasn't a doctor. The Cassidy Brothers are notorious villains. I suggest if you haven't already you clear the ward of visitors and get them out of the hospital as soon as possible.'

'Yes, Sister,' I replied as she hung up.

I gulped. 'Freddy, we've got work to do. Come on.'

Staff Nurse was already on to it before I had the chance to pass on the Casualty Sister's message. 'Ah, Mr Cassidy, we meet again,' she said to the tall, thin man in a sharp suit holding the little boy. He was standing between two shorter, stockier men with broken noses and cauliflower ears, practically identical and snarling like guard dogs. 'And is this the latest addition?' Staff asked calmly.

'Yeah, Billy's my youngest. Finally a boy after all them girls, you'll be glad to hear. Burnt his arse on electric fire, silly little sod. Here you go, Nurse,' he said, handing the bare-bottom child over.

'Nurse Hill, please go run a very cold bath immediately and I will bring Billy in directly,' instructed Staff Nurse Lennard. 'Gentleman, bay one is empty if you'd wait in there with Doctor,' she ordered. I saw Freddy involuntarily shake his head as he nervously followed the men into the bay.

Staff Nurse was swiftly on my heels. Poor Billy Cassidy was only a baby. He should have been sobbing but he was past all tears now and just quivering. We lowered him into the icy cold bath and gave him little sips of water as we submerged him until the heat of the burn had cooled off. He soon revived and wanted to get out of the freezing cold water, but we had to keep him in there for ten minutes until we could be sure it had done its work on the burn. When I lifted Billy out of the bath there were two bright red burn lines across his bottom.

'Fetch the non-adhesive lint to dry him with and we'll take him into Dr MacDonald,' Staff told me. I wrapped Billy gently in a towel and carried him through to bay one.

The Cassidy men were playing cards on the little table in the bay. I almost laughed at the sight of these huge men sitting on tiny little chairs dealing out a hand. Freddy was hovering near the door. The brothers ignored him; he was no threat to them. Staff Nurse lowered the side of a cot and I gently placed Billy on the towel so Freddy could examine him. The Cassidy Brothers stopped playing cards and watched the doctor very closely. Freddy's hands were shaking slightly as he looked at the burn marks. Billy's father, Charlie Cassidy, got to his feet and stood over Freddy.

'Mind how you touch my boy. I know what you posh fellas are like,' he warned. The pitbull-like twins snorted at this and Freddy gave a nervous laugh as well, which didn't go down well with Charlie Cassidy, who grabbed the young houseman's arms and said, 'You think I'm joking, Posh Boy?'

Freddy was so scared he couldn't get a word out. Luckily for him Staff Nurse Lennard came to his rescue. 'We'll use a non-adhesive lint to dry the skin, apply some soothing cream and put a nappy on the boy before he has an accident. Would you recommend a strong painkiller administered in droplets every four hours, Doctor?'

'Yes, Staff Nurse, quite right,' said Freddy, trying to keep the tremble out of his voice. And then he scarpered, leaving us to deal with the Cassidy Brothers. Staff Nurse started to fill in Billy's chart, seeing as Freddy had taken off without a by your leave.

'How did Billy come to sit on the electric fire, Mr Cassidy?'

'It's his mother's fault really. I was playing cards with my brothers and this other fella, what's his name, Jacky?'

'Manderville,' answered one of the brothers.

'Yes, Manderville. He's from South Africa and he keeps complaining it's so cold, see. So Johnny here, he puts on an electric fire to keep us all warm. Well, we're only a few hands in and the boy's mother turns up. Says she's got to leave him with me on account of she's got to go into hospital. Silly mare's up the duff again and says it's her time and how she wants me to have Billy while she goes for a little lie down in the Mothers' Hospital. I says to her, "Can't you leave him with your ma or your sister or someone? I'm busy." She replies all uppity, "My sister's picking up the girls from school and my ma's coming with me to the hospital." Well I ask you, so she just leaves him in his pram and takes off. Before we know it he's making a right old fuss, so we takes him out of the pram and give him the spare deck of cards and a packet of Ready Salted and a bottle of pop to have under the table while we get on with our game. I got up to go for a piss and left Tweedledum and Tweedledee in charge of young Billy, only they're too busy to watch over their nephew – my son and heir – and let him burn his behind on the electric fire. So I put him in the motor and gets him here lickety-split.'

'Don't blame us, Charlie,' said one of the brothers, getting up from his tiny chair.

'Did I say you could speak? Haven't you done enough for one day?'

'I'm not a bloody nursemaid. It's not my fault your missus can't take care of all them kids you keep getting on her,' retaliated Jacky Cassidy, coming nose to chin with his taller sibling.

'You want to shut your mouth, Jacky Boy, before I shuts it for you,' said Charlie.

'Brains you may have, but you're no good with your fists, Charlie,' teased his brother, and then they actually started having a punch-up. Open-mouthed toddlers started popping up at the window panes to watch these men brawling like hooligans. Babies were screaming and nurses were running all over the place trying to get the children back in their beds and out of harm's way. Fortunately, Staff Nurse Lennard had seen to it that all visitors were shown out while we were giving Billy his cold bath, so at least there were no parents to witness this débâcle. After each of the brothers had laid a few punches, the third brother sluggishly got to his feet and separated them.

'Leave it out now, you two. Jacky, can't you see Charlie's worried about Billy?' said Johnny Cassidy. 'You're upsetting the little lad.'

I was holding Billy tightly to my chest, fearful of him getting caught up in the skirmish. Charlie Cassidy smiled at me and ran his hands through his dark hair, smoothing it out and dusting off his suit. 'Go and wait outside, the pair of you. I won't be long,' he told his brothers. Obediently Johnny and Jacky Cassidy got to their feet and took their leave.

'Visiting time is long over,' said Staff Nurse, 'and I'll expect you'll want to see how your wife is getting on.'

'It's her fifth, Nurse. Must be all over by now. But you're right enough, I'll stop by the Mothers' Hospital and tell her what a neglectful mare she is, and when she comes out she can pick up Billy as well, all right?'

'Very well, Mr Cassidy. We'll take care of Billy.'

'I know you will. God bless Mr Churchill for setting up the NHS.'

My mouth dropped open and I was just about to correct him when I saw Staff Nurse Lennard give me a small shake of the head. Mr Cassidy gave me a wink and left not a moment too soon. I didn't see Freddy again for the rest of my shift. Too scared to come back, I suspected.

9

I had a very rare morning off and yet here I was up to my elbows in felt and ribbons in the Infants Ward laundry room. We had little drawstring bags made by the ladies of the parish, which Maddox and I were stuffing with Christmas presents for the children's party at St Barnabas that afternoon. Lined up before us were tangerines, a jar full of sixpences, sugar mice and chocolate coins – the booty for each bag to be given out after a puppet show and tea by the vicar, who would be dressed as Father Christmas. We'd nearly finished and Maddox had written out a little label for each child so there wouldn't be a muddle about which bag belonged to who after they'd been opened and then inevitably discarded.

'Who's left?' asked Maddox as she finished a label with a flourish.

'Just Annie Donnelly and Flo Lindell,' I replied, checking the list.

Maddox wrote out Flo's label and passed it to me to be tied onto a red felt bag with a green ribbon. 'Bother, I've run out of labels,' she said. 'I'll just pop to Sister's office and get another. I won't be two ticks.'

Maddox scurried off and I started to put the gift bags into a large cardboard box to take over to the church. The children were going to have such a lovely time. Mums and dads were allowed to come for the party, so some of them had a whole afternoon together to look forward to as well as a visit from Father Christmas.

'And have you been naughty or nice?' said a familiar plummy voice rather too close behind me.

Freddy had crept in. 'Oh, it's you. I haven't seen you for a while,' I said coolly.

Freddy cleared his throat. 'Well, no. I've been in male surgical.' Truth be told he'd gone to the hospital secretary, an old golfing buddy of his father, and got moved for fear of running into the Cassidy Brothers again. 'I've just been so busy, but I've missed you, Sarah.' I didn't reply. 'And I've got two tickets to see "The Black and White Minstrel Show".'

'I wouldn't see that show. Not with you, not with anybody. It's disgusting.'

'Steady on, Sarah. It's just a bit of fun. I didn't buy the tickets, they were given to me by the hospital secretary. It's not really my cup of tea, either – bit old fashioned. What about the back seat of the Odeon instead?' He leered, getting rather too close as I picked up the last of the sixpences to put into Annie's bag. Freddy's eyes suddenly flitted to the sixpence.

'Hang on,' he said taking the coin from me. 'That's a Victorian sixpence.'

'So?' I said, snatching it back.

'It's valuable,' he said, his eyes still fixed on the coin.

'Well, that'll be nice for Annie.'

'What do you say you give me that sixpence and I'll give you a nice shiny one for Annie from my pocket instead,' he said, his hands searching through his trouser pockets for a replacement coin.

'No, Freddy. It's Annie's sixpence. You can't take it from her.'

'She'll never know.'

'That's not the point. We'll know.'

'I really don't see what the problem is, Sarah.'

'The problem is you are despicable and want to rob a little girl of her money. Get out, Freddy, and don't bother me ever again,' I told him in a steady, calm voice. He just huffed and shoved past Maddox as she came back in with the final label.

'What's wrong with him?' she asked.

'Who cares, but I don't think he'll be bothering me again,' I said as I wrote out the final label for Annie Donnelly and popped her Victorian sixpence into the drawstring bag. I would ensure this was delivered from Father Christmas myself.

Appleton had already gone over with a clutch of toddlers, all holding hands in a line between her and Pearl, for the puppet show. Sister Skinflint, in a more jovial mood than usual, was seen pushing a little boy in a wheelchair out of the ward, leading a chorus of 'Good King Wenceslas' with the older children. There was just Patel and I left, and we were getting ready to take over the older babies who were well enough to go to enjoy the carols and present opening. Staff Nurse Lennard volunteered to remain with the younger babies; she did not celebrate Christmas.

As we crossed over the road to St Barnabas I saw Mrs Edwards running down the street with little Georgie in her arms looking panic stricken. I hurriedly passed the baby I was holding to Patel to take into the church and rushed to Mrs Edwards. Georgie was barely breathing; he was red in the face and not responding to her cries. I felt his face and he was so hot.

'How long has he been like this, Mrs Edwards?'

'I don't know. I've just come home and found him like this,' she cried.

'Quick, let's get him straight to Casualty.' I took her by the arm, guiding her through the traffic and into the hospital. As soon as we entered Casualty I saw Charge Nurse Andrews behind the desk. I ran to him.

'Twelve-month-old baby, reoccurring bronchitis, non-responsive, high temperature. He's very floppy and I can't get a response.'

'Quick, into cubicle one. I'll bleep the paediatrician,' instructed the Charge Nurse. His team flew into action, taking little Georgie off Mrs Edwards and screening him off from view. In minutes Dr Warren was there and I waited the other side of the curtain with Mrs Edwards as she trembled and shook. It must have only been about three minutes but it felt like three hours as we waited in silence, and then we heard Georgie cry.

'Thank God,' cried Mrs Edwards as she hugged me to her.

I patted her back. 'Everything will be well.'

'This time,' she sniffed. 'But what about next time? That place, it'll be the death of us all.'

Nurse Kaur emerged from behind the cubicle curtain holding little Georgie. His mother flew to him and kissed his head.

'Good job,' Charge Nurse Andrews told me. 'We'll take it from here.'

My blood was pumping; I stormed out of the hospital and to St Barnabas to find Sister Nivern. She'd done nothing to help those children, nothing at all. How could she stand there in a church at Christmas knowing she'd not lifted a finger to help two babies who could die if they didn't get help soon. I marched into the hall. All the children were laughing at Mr Punch chasing the dog who had nicked his sausages. Sister was standing next to the vicar's wife, enjoying the show with a cup of tea.

'Sister, may I have a word please,' I asked, trying to keep my voice calm and steady. The vicar's wife tactfully excused herself.

'Ah, Nurse Hill. I thought you'd abandoned your post,' tittered Sister Nivern.

'I just had to rush Georgie Edwards to Casualty with breathing difficulties.'

'Who?' she asked absentmindedly, her focus still on the puppet show.

'One of the babies in the steam tents last month,' I reminded her.

'Ah, yes. Well, bronchitis, it does happen.'

'You said you'd speak to the Lady Almoner about finding them better living conditions.'

'Did I?'

'Yes, you did.'

Sister Nivern now fixed her gaze on me. 'I don't seem to recall anything of the kind. I wouldn't bother the Lady Almoner with a case like that, not when we have children without parents that need homes.'

'But Sister, Georgie Edwards could have died today. His home is making him and his cousin ill. I think both the mothers are depressed. It is costing the State far more to treat them than it would be to properly house them.'

'Nurse Hill, you come from a nice family and are a well-brought-up young lady with eight O-levels. I don't expect you to understand why the lower orders live how they do, but that is how it is. That is how it will always be. Give them an indoor bathroom and they'd keep coal in it,' she snickered.

'But Sister …' I tried again.

'But nothing. Not another word, Nurse. That is how things are, now get on with your work,' she informed me as she turned away and walked over to join Matron, who had come to observe the festivities.

I felt powerless. I couldn't help them. I wasn't even a proper student nurse yet. I could only nurse the babies again and be kind to the mothers, but it wasn't enough. Maybe Gerald or the vicar would know what to do. Surely someone would know how to put this right, but nobody did, not then. I slipped away into the church and prayed to be shown a way to help them. And I was, but not that Christmas.

When I returned to the hall the children were lined up receiving their Christmas presents from Father Christmas. Annie Donnelly was just hopping onto his knee to whisper what she wanted to find in her stocking on Christmas morning. I saw Mr Donnelly, the mechanic, watching his daughter with pride.

'What do you think she'll ask for?' I said.

'Not a doll and a pram like all the other girls,' he smiled. 'She's been after a fire engine in the toy shop window on Mare Street but it's a bit too expensive.'

Annie rushed over, munching on her sugar mouse already. 'Look Daddy, and I got a sixpence too.'

'Can I see your sixpence please, Annie?' I asked. She nodded and handed it up to me. I pretended to inspect it. 'Mr Donnelly, I think if you take this sixpence to a coin dealer you might want to also visit a certain shop in Mare Street afterwards,' I told him, pointing out the date engraved on the coin.

Mr Donnelly stared at it and his face lit up. 'Thank you, Nurse. I think that's a very good idea. Merry Christmas,' he beamed.

1969 was almost over and those first three months at Hackney had taught me more than all the private schools had in over a decade. As I rushed that evening to catch the train to Wales for a Hill Family Christmas I knew I wasn't the same girl who'd set off in her father's chauffeur-driven car at the end of the summer. I knew that life was harsh, that I couldn't fix everything, but I also knew that I could make a difference here. Hackney had already become my home and I couldn't wait for the New Year and for my Preliminary Nurse Training to begin.

10

I looked at the empty seat tucked neatly under the wooden desk next to me. A month into Preliminary Training School, or PTS as we called it, and every single student nurse knew it was a grave misdemeanour to be late for one of Sister Connors's classes. My friend Daniels was never late, and it was almost nine o'clock in the morning. It was very hard to find a plausible excuse for tardiness given the luxury of, firstly, the classes not starting till nine and, secondly, the school being practically next door to the nurses' home.

'Have you seen Daniels?' I whispered to Bonnett sitting at the desk behind me.

'Not since Friday when she went into giggles during Sister Powell's bed bathing demonstration,' replied Bonnett, rolling her eyes.

'What do you expect? Everyone knows they can't keep time,' said the overtly priggish student nurse sitting at the desk in front of me.

'I wasn't talking to you, Prendergast,' I hissed back.

Prendergast swivelled round to face the blackboard. She was sitting in the middle desk of the front row – *teacher's pet*.

Over the last few weeks since starting PTS I had come to loathe the sight of her dull brown curly head, her stubby features and most of all her abhorrent views, always expressed in clipped, unnatural tones in an attempt to hide that she was a coal merchant's daughter from Shropshire. Prendergast liked to talk about hunting, dates with doctors and how the Labour government was opening up Britain to immigration and with it ruin and pestilence. This despite the fact that in this classroom it was the white girls who were the minority – there only being me, her and five Irish girls out of the fifty students in the class – but I think this fuelled her sense of outrage and supposed superiority.

Sister Connors strode in and started to rearrange the desk which she shared with the other Nurse Tutor, the recently arrived Sister Powell. They were like chalk and cheese. Sister Connors was from a hardworking Irish Catholic family; small and wiry, she liked to have everything in its proper place, preferred you to be silent unless spoken to and took the calling of nursing as solemnly as a bride of Christ. Sister Powell on the other hand would waft in late, her red hair loosely tied and her large hazel eyes still glazed from a Bohemian party the night before. Sister Powell preferred to gently lead us through our lessons, using questions and discussion rather than the long-serving Sister Connors's teaching method of no-nonsense instruction with a telling off if you made a mistake.

Sister Connors wrinkled up her nose in disgust as she cleared away Sister Powell's tea cup and dropped empty humbug wrappers into the bin. She sighed at the flowery handwriting that hadn't been wiped from the blackboard since Friday, and it was at this moment, while Sister Connors's back was turned, that Daniels expertly slipped into the classroom.

'Where have you been?' I whispered.

'I need you to do me a favour,' she said, unperturbed, keeping her Tobagonian equanimity and ignoring my question completely. 'Are you doing anything tonight, Hill?'

'No, why?'

'I met this boy on the bus. His name's Adam. He's asked me on a date tonight and he wants to bring his brother. So I need you to go on a double date with me.'

'I don't know …'

'Oh, come on now, Hill. You know how lonely I've been since I've come here. Now a nice boy has asked me out on a date. It's just a bit of fun.'

'I've got work to do. There's mid-term tests coming up, you know …'

'Work, work, work,' Daniels interrupted my excuses. 'Don't you know it's bad for your health not to take a little break now and again? All work and no play makes Sarah Hill a dull girl.'

I scowled slightly. It was true; since we'd started PTS I'd had my nose in a book most of the time. I was so thrilled to no longer be just an extra pair of hands and be a proper student nurse. But despite my three months on Infants

Ward, I'd found the real challenge was putting the theory into practice on the ward. A few girls had already dropped out after being faced with dressings, injections and bed baths. Nursing isn't for the faint hearted.

Daniels gave me huge puppy dog eyes and pouted her lower lip. Maybe a night out would do me good. I relented.

'All right, then. What are we doing?'

'I said we'd meet them at Leicester Square at seven o'clock.'

'What are we doing?' I repeated. God, was I going to have to drag every scrap of information out of her?

'Odeon to see *Butch Cassidy and the Sundance Kid*,' she whispered back.

Sister Connors spun round. 'Student Nurse Daniels, is your social calendar in order? Would you mind if I started the lesson?' she asked through a forced smile.

I slunk down in my seat. A date I didn't want, Sister Connors glaring at me – not a great start to the week.

After the credits started to roll, our foursome gathered up coats, scarves and gloves and sailed out of the Leicester Square Odeon on a wave of excitement, all humming 'Raindrops Keep Falling on My Head'. Daniels and her date Andy's humming soon turned into heady singing, having partaken of a few pints in the pub before we went into the cinema. I had waited with Alex, a stranger, outside the smoke-filled bar as he'd said it was too crowded and he'd rather just talk outside. Even though it was the end of

January and madness to be standing around street corners, for some reason I found I couldn't say no to him and happily nattered while he listened intently, both of us stamping our feet and hugging ourselves to keep warm against the cold night air, both filled with the anticipation of seeing Robert Redford.

As we merged with the crowd, Daniels and Andy strode out confidently ahead, laughing, walking hip to hip, whispering in each other's ears suggestively, her hand in the pocket of his jeans, Andy's arm wrapped tightly round my friend's waist. Both their heads were a mass of black curls that intertwined when they kissed. I watched the delicate way her dark brown hand softly stroked his pale white cheek, and then looked away, embarrassed.

Alex and I followed Daniels and Andy at a distance through the throng of pleasure seekers, walking close together but not touching, talking quietly. Our pauses were filled with shy smiles and widening eyes. I felt light and happy and safe. The night sky was illuminated by the rainbow-coloured lights of London's West End – we weren't in Hackney any more.

As we made our way past the tube station and down St Martin's Lane, Alex asked in a voice so quiet that only I could hear him. 'Did you like the film, Sarah?' He spoke like everything was a secret between just us two – it was intoxicating.

'I loved it,' I replied. 'Especially the bit with the bike when she rode on his handlebars,' I giggled.

He grinned, 'Me too,' and I felt his hand brush against mine. A rush of excitement ran through me. I let my hand brush back against his.

Alex was tall and slim, his hair was blond and curly and needed a trim – it kept falling into his pale blue eyes, making him blink behind his glasses.

We wandered through the lions in Trafalgar Square. Sitting on the fountain was a group of teddy boys. As we went past them, by now in a tighter foursome so we wouldn't lose each other in the crowds, they started to make monkey noises and jump up and down furiously.

'Oi, mate. Why don't you take your monkey back to the jungle where you found her,' shouted one of them at Andy, who froze on the spot and glared at them, his eyes burning with rage.

Alex put a steady hand on his non-identical twin's arm. 'Don't,' he implored of his brother.

'Do you want to come over here without your mates and say that?' shouted Andy, filled with fury and ready for a fight.

Daniels didn't say anything. She shook her head sadly, her eyes blinking as she forced the tears, the hurt and the shame to stay locked away inside. I took her hand and tried to lead her away; I wanted to get her out of this. The teddy boy, with his greased-back hair greying at the temples and about the ears, smugly stayed where he was with his mates. 'Stay where I am, thanks,' he sneered at us, grinning like a gargoyle. 'Wouldn't want to catch something. When you've finished with your gollywog get yourself down the doctor's,' he laughed as his friends exploded with mirth.

Andy marched towards the gang, pushing up his jacket sleeves.

'Stop,' shouted Alex. Half way between us and the gang Andy stopped in his tracks at this command from his shy, quiet sibling. He turned back to face us. 'They are nothing but ignorant, sad men,' Alex said. 'Nothing better to do than hang around on a freezing cold night and harass kids. How's getting your head kicked in going to help her? They want a fight – they want to upset her,' he explained in a low, steady voice. 'Don't let them do it.'

Andy came back to us and smiled softly at Daniels. He put his fingertips to her downward chin and lifted her head. 'You're so beautiful,' he told her and then he kissed her slowly, not fervently like before but tenderly.

Andy led my lovely friend by the hand through the square towards Whitehall. Alex and I followed. I didn't say anything about what had happened but I was so impressed. Alex was different. I hadn't met anyone like him before; just being with him filled me with a quiet confidence that I was safe in his hands. He wasn't fumbling and forceful like the Freddies of this world I'd previously encountered.

We stood together at the bus stop by Westminster stamping our feet to keep warm, Daniels and Andy kissing, Alex and I side by side as we waited for the bus to take us back to Hackney.

'Have you ever been to the House of Commons, Sarah?' he asked. We'd been discussing politics at length, and particularly the debate around nurses' pay that was filling the column inches of the newspapers.

'No, but I'm going there to hear the final debate on nurses' pay on my afternoon off next week,' I answered. Maddox had insisted I accompany her as she was the nurses' home principal campaigner for the 'Raise the Roof' campaign to improve pay.

'Would you like me to come with you?' he asked, keeping his eyes firmly fixed on his scuffed shoes as he kicked the frozen ground nervously.

'I'd love that,' I said. 'I'll give you the number of the pay phone at the nurses' home. Will you ring me?'

'Of course I will,' he said, as I rapidly scribbled my number on the back of a receipt with a blunt pencil from my handbag.

Alex grinned as he pocketed the paper and our bus drew up. Daniels leapt on the back of the Routemaster, waving to Andy and blowing him kisses. Alex took my hand as I stepped up onto the back of the bus. Daniels and I rushed up to the top deck to get a better view of the boys as the bus pulled away so we could wave. As Alex disappeared from view I felt my heart do a little leap of longing and hope. 'Oh, no,' I thought. 'What does that mean?' But I already knew. I was going to fall in love with him.

11

The first ward I was let loose on during PTS was Male Surgical under the excellent tutelage of Charge Nurse Davis or Daddy Davis as we affectionately called him. He'd already insisted that I wear my black-rimmed spectacles at all times and I begrudgingly agreed with him – I couldn't see how much fluid was left in the drips without them, and on the Male Surgical Ward there were a lot of drips. Daddy Davis was tall with a ruddy complexion. His white tunic cut at elbow length revealed muscular forearms built up no doubt from the constant lifting, and his black hair was thinning in middle age. His nose was sharp but his eyes were always kind. Daddy Davis would tell us often, 'Be good to the patients and I will be good to you,' and he really meant it. He guided us with gentle and confident instruction. He led us through taking out stitches and giving injections with care and compassion to the patient, resulting in both patient and student coming out of preliminary training mostly unscathed. During visiting hours he'd often give us an impromptu lesson, perhaps on the male urinary system by drawing the kidneys or bladder on a wooden board that covered the bath tub. He'd tell us, 'Don't be afraid to ask questions. Sometimes a question can make the difference between life and death.'

During my tea round I was called away from my trolley by Bertie Lamptey, a car salesman who was in to have his kidney stones out that afternoon.

'Here, Nurse. I'm Taters in the Mould in here. Close that window would you,' he called out, and I noticed the whole ward pricked up their ears.

'All right, Mr Lamptey. We don't want you to get too excited before your operation, do we?' I said.

He had a chuckle and gave a wink to old Mr Mason in the bed next to him as I hitched up my skirt and climbed onto the huge radiator underneath the window nearest his bed. I stretched up to try and reach the high window but as I am only five foot one and a half it was a bit of a struggle. As my fingers fumbled to unlock the catch my skirt rode up high on the leg, revealing the threepenny bit I was using to keep my black stockings up until I could afford to buy some new suspenders.

'You're the one who's getting him too excited, Nurse,' called out Mr Mason, laughing with Mr Lamptey and all rest of the ward. Matron came through the doors with Daddy Davis to peals of laughter and cheers.

'Nurse, get down at once. What is all this excitement about?'

'I was just opening a window, Matron,' I replied, quickly jumping down and straightening out my uniform.

The men stifled their laughter – they didn't want to get on the wrong side of Matron.

'Mr Lamptey should be prepped for his operation by now,' snapped Matron.

'Nurse Hill and I are just going to do it now, Matron,' Daddy Davis informed her, stepping forward to screen off the bed. Matron carried on with her round, asking each patient how they were today, as she did every day without fail.

'Right, Hill, fetch the trolley with the canvas sheet and we'll get Mr Lamptey prepped and off to theatre,' instructed Daddy Davis.

I dashed off to get the trolley and returned eager to show him just how much I'd learnt. I confidently injected Mr Lamptey with his pre-med into his thigh and chatted to him while we waited for the drug to kick in. Everything changed though when I asked him to get onto the trolley to go down to theatre. At first I thought he hadn't heard me say, 'Hop on,' but then I realised he was ignoring me. I had to firmly coax my reluctant patient out of his bed, and just when I thought I'd finally got him comfortable on the trolley he sat up bolt upright, his brow furrowed with fear.

Mr Lamptey shouted in a terrified voice, 'I'm not going. Get my trousers. I'm going home.' He sprang up with the intention of making a run for it, but the pre-med he'd received during prep was making him woozy and uncoordinated, though it felt to me he still had all his strength as I struggled to keep him on the trolley. Just when I thought I'd finally pacified him and he was lying down calmly and ready to go down to theatre, he jumped up like a jack-in-the-box and shouted that he wasn't going to let anyone cut him open. I was starting to despair when Daddy Davis came to my rescue. With quiet confidence he pulled the curtain closed and spoke to Mr Lamptey kindly but firmly. I nervously waited on the other side, the eyes of every man on the ward on me, making me feel even more uncomfortable than when they were taking a cheeky look at my stockings.

'Come on, old chap, keep it together for that young nurse,' I heard Daddy Davis whisper to our reluctant patient. 'She's just begun her training and you don't want her to give up because of you, do you?'

And like a lamb Mr Lamptey got onto the trolley and gave me a weak little wink as he was wheeled off by the hospital porters. Just then Matron reappeared looking like something was on her mind.

'Cutting it a little fine for theatre, aren't we?' I heard her say to Daddy Davis as I made up Mr Lamptey's crumpled bed. Daddy Davis smiled at her; he knew she didn't mean anything by it.

'Can I help you with anything, Matron?' he asked.

'Yes. Earlier,' she hesitated. Matron never hesitated. 'Nurse Hill on the radiator?'

'Yes?' he asked, just slightly raising one eyebrow. Clearly Matron didn't understand what all the fuss was about; this was out of her field of expertise. 'Black stockings, Matron,' Daddy Davis explained with a wry smile.

'Black stockings?'

'Men do rather like them. Gets them a bit excited.'

'But they are regulation. I insist all the nurses wear them.'
Daddy Davis just smiled and waited for the penny or rather
the threepenny bit to drop. 'Ah, I see. Thank you, Charge
Nurse Davis, you've given me something to think about,'
she said, scuttling off in a most un-Matron-like hurry.

I chuckled just a little to myself and thought about what
a laugh we'd have when I told the girls about Matron getting
all of a fluster over nylons. She clearly hadn't been around
men much outside of the hospital if she didn't know a little
thing like that. Even a convent boarding school girl like me
seemed to have more experience of the opposite sex than
old Matron, I thought, as Daddy Davis called me over to Mr
Mason's bed.

'Hill, Mr Mason's wound needs dressing. You'll need to
use ribbon gauze, a solution of eusol and paraffin to pack it.'

I bustled off to get the equipment, eager once more to
show how much I'd learnt. Then I remembered just what
poor Mr Mason's wound was and stopped right in my tracks.
He was in to heal a gaping hole in his scrotum which had
resulted from untreated syphilis. I flushed scarlet as I gathered up the equipment and laid out my trolley. Now who's
the unworldly one, Sarah?

But it turned out my embarrassment was nothing
compared to Mr Mason's discomfort. He never complained
once as I changed his dressing, which must have been very
painful. He had so much to put up with – the horrid disease

meant he had to have a catheter which drained into a urinary bag, as well as a whole host of problems. I determined to follow Daddy Davis's example and do my best to show him the respect and care he deserved. It proved to be an uncomfortable but valuable lesson.

Only a couple of hours after Mr Lamptey returned from theatre with his kidney stones successfully removed, he was back to his normal cheeky chappy self. Just as I was about to come off duty, eager to get back to the nurses' home to get ready for my trip to the House of Commons, he beckoned me to his bedside once more.

'Here, Nurse,' he called out.

'Yes, Mr Lamptey?' I asked. He'd better not be expecting me to get up on that radiator, I thought. I'd had quite enough of that sort of thing for one day.

'Here you are,' he said, putting his business card into my hand. 'You ever need a motor, come and see me and I'll see you right,' he insisted, tapping his nose.

'I'll take you up on that when I pass my test,' I said cheerily as I pocketed the card and waved him goodbye.

I looked at my little upside-down nurse's watch. Oh, I really had to get a move on if I was going to get to Westminster on time. Maddox would be furious if we were late and missed the debate. As I strode through the lobby of the nurses' home a group of girls were gathered round the notice board sniggering. Wade chortling the loudest of them all.

'What's all this?' I asked, curiosity getting the better of me.

'It's a notice from Matron,' Wade explained. 'Orders that no nurse is to wear black stockings, starting from tomorrow. Neutral ones are now the regulation colour.'

'Well, thank heaven for that,' I laughed. 'I'm sick of black stockings, they show every tiny ladder. We'll save a packet.'

'I know. I wonder what's changed old Matron's mind?'

I shrugged. My story would have to wait till bedtime. I needed to get ready for my date, or rather the big debate.

Maddox had brought a huge placard with her saying 'Fair Pay for Nurses' in big red painted letters. She held it high all the way on the bus from Hackney to Westminster and didn't give a damn as she knocked her fellow passengers about the head with it. I was so embarrassed as we trundled along with commuters and pleasure seekers out for a night up West, but there was Maddox excitedly talking about her vigil with the lobbyists the previous week. On the night Daniels and I were out with Alex and Andy, Maddox had been petitioning MPs to improve nurses' pay. She may have been a bit over the top but her heart was in the right place. When we eventually arrived at Parliament Square on the last Tuesday of January 1970 it was long past eight o'clock. I squinted anxiously into the gloom to see if Alex was still there. To my relief I saw him waiting by a lamp on the small patch of lawn opposite Westminster. He must have been frozen, poor thing.

It was only a week since our first date but I'd met up with him three times since then just to go for a walk when I got off duty, and he telephoned the nurses' home every single night. It felt like he'd always be a part of things. We had our first kiss walking along the river holding hands on a chilly evening, our breath hanging around in frozen puffs of air as we talked rapidly about plans for the future.

Alex worked in a bank but he hated it. He was desperate to get out of his father's maisonette in Stamford Hill, where he, Andy and their older brother Pete all lived on top of one another – four grown men in a two-bed flat. He told me that it wasn't much of a home since his mother had died four years ago, when he was sixteen, just before he took his O-levels. And now his dad had taken up with a fancy woman who was round all the time and Alex hadn't taken to her one bit. Her name was Margie and she was loud, far too loud for someone reserved like Alex. Margie drank and smoked – always wore too much make-up and strong perfume, and told dirty jokes that made poor Alex squirm. His mother, he told me, had been slight and blonde and quiet, and only really spoke up when she had something important to say. He missed her terribly, I could tell.

I didn't say much about my own family; just gave the statistics and none of the details. Alex told me how much he dreamed of leaving London and living in the countryside with no neighbours, just chickens and maybe a goat where he could grow his own food and be his own man. 'I'd need the right girl to do it with,' he whispered in a low voice as we'd passed the shadow of St Paul's Cathedral one night. Was I the right girl then? I'd been trying my whole life to get out of the country to the city and he'd been dreaming of the opposite escape route. I almost laughed, but I didn't want Alex to think I was laughing at him and not tell me any more. I wanted him to tell me everything.

Now, I trekked across the grass towards my new boyfriend in my navy reefer jacket, getting mud on my white boots. Alex was taking pictures of Westminster Abbey with his precious Nikon F camera, lighting up the small patch of lawn with the flash as he clicked away. As soon as I caught his eye we both broke out into big smiles. I felt my stomach do a little summersault at the sight of him smiling at me and then he quickly lifted his camera and took my photo. I hurried over to him just to get a few seconds on our own before Maddox caught up. She was trudging after me prac-tising the chant she'd composed out loud during our bus journey. Alex seized the opportunity to kiss me swiftly but sweetly. His hair needed a comb, I could see his open-necked shirt under his dark grey jacket, and his jeans were scuffed where they'd been dragging on the ground.

'Let's get a shot of you two with the placard,' said Alex as he lifted the camera which was hanging around his neck up to his eye once more. Obediently Maddox and I stood together with Westminster Palace as our backdrop. 'Just stand a little closer together,' he directed.

In the distance I could see a police constable storming over the grass towards us, attracted by the light of Alex's camera. 'What do you think you are doing?' he shouted at Alex.

'I'm just taking the girls' picture before we go in to hear the debate.'

The policeman, who was now on top of us, pushed Alex and pulled his camera right off his neck, deliberately breaking the cord as he did it. 'I know your sort,' the policeman sneered. 'You young layabouts think you can do whatever you like. Hellraisers, the lot of you.'

'Can I have my camera back, please?' asked Alex in a low, calm voice.

'I think I might keep it, get it developed – evidence. See what you're really up to,' he said, pompously rocking back and forth on his heels, passing Alex's precious camera back and forth roughly between his hands.

'If you feel that's necessary, Constable,' replied Alex.

'You've got no right to do that,' I shouted at the policeman, angry and hurt that he should treat Alex so roughly when he'd done nothing to deserve it.

'What's a nice girl like you doing with a hippy like him? Your dad know you're out?' the policeman condescended.

'Trust the fuzz to be sexist pigs,' shouted Maddox unhelpfully.

'Leave it,' said Alex. 'If you want the camera take it, only give me a ticket so I know which station to pick it up from.'

He eyeballed Alex and chucked the camera at him. 'Your sort's not worth the paperwork,' he sneered and went off to harass a group of hippies gathered on another part of the square.

'Why didn't you stand up for yourself?' I cried out.

'And give the man what he wants? He wanted to pick a fight and then arrest me, Sarah.'

'Did he?' I asked, looking up at him, the hot tears that had been pricking at my eyes, threatening to fall, fading back in relief.

'Will you two stop messing about or we won't get a seat in the gallery for the debate,' scolded Maddox. We turned on our heels and hurried to join the queue into Westminster.

We were packed in tight in the Strangers' Gallery, elbow to elbow with our fellow NHS militants, and across the chasm of the chamber that divided the House of Commons sat rows of journalists – all of us ready to hear the fate of nurses' purses as debated by the politicians. I hoped we did get a pay rise; it was a real challenge stretching the money out each month. I was lucky. I could always write home and ask for a few bob, though I never did.

The chamber was much smaller than I'd expected. I cast my eye over the House – other than a few familiar faces on the front bench, the men and few women who ran our country were largely unknown to me. At just past nine o'clock in the evening, I couldn't believe how many of them looked like the wine had got the better of them. One or two were unashamedly napping as they waited for the Speaker to call order.

Eventually the Speaker made his dramatic entrance up the steps to his bench. Dressed in a black gown with a stiff white shirt and stockings, he even had shiny buckles on his shoes, and to top off his ensemble he wore a wig, making him look more like a judge than a politician. He waited for the chatter to subside until he had the attention of the House and began. We had to sit through some boring drivel until the nurses' pay debate started. Maddox and her friends had taken up residence in the gallery for the last week, so knew now to come with sweets secreted in their pockets to ease the tedium. I started to sympathise with some of the old MPs who were dozing, as I felt my own eyes begin to tire after the busy day on Male Surgical. Maddox nudged me hard and I refocused and heard the Speaker say,

'I remind the House that this is the fifth of twenty-five debates that are to take place during the night. Reasonably brief speeches will help.'

'Hallelujah. But twenty-five debates at this time of night? It explains a lot, doesn't it?' whispered Alex. 'We can sneak out after this one, can't we? Or we'll miss the last bus home.'

'I hope so,' I whispered back as the Speaker invited the honourable Member for Fife West to take the floor.

Mr William Hamilton MP stood up. He was flamboyantly dressed in tartan trousers, and began his speech with all the formality of a Westminster politician, taking at least fifteen minutes to say something that without all the posturing could have been said in three. 'The House will recall that, on

2 December last, I initiated a debate on precisely the question of the nursing profession ...'

'I wonder how much the House does recall?' whispered Alex. 'They all seem to like the sound of their own voice regardless of which side they are on.'

I smiled and tuned back into Mr Hamilton. '... the dissatisfaction of the nursing profession with its lot has intensified. Morale has declined, and militancy, if of a genteel character, has increased. The decline in morale is not caused solely by low pay. It is partly due to a lack of efficient organisation by the nurses themselves ...'

'Who's he calling genteel?' I said to Maddox.

'You, probably,' she mocked. The one time Maddox made a joke, and it was at my expense.

'Secondly,' continued Mr Hamilton, 'the career structure of the nursing profession is unsatisfactory and it seems that the implementation of the Salmon Committee proposals on this matter is proceeding very slowly.'

'Bloody Salmonisation – it's a disgrace,' I spat out. Alex looked rather surprised but I couldn't stop myself. Surely anyone could see that replacing Matron with administrative managers wasn't going to work. No one knew what was going on in the hospital like Matron. She might not be my favourite person in the world but you couldn't deny her magnificence. She knew every patient by name, and their condition, and when she asked them how they were every single day she listened, and heaven help you if they complained about their care. I didn't believe for one minute an administrator in an office was going to do that – how would they actually know what was going on in the hospital? I wasn't the only one who'd seen red at the mention of Salmon as a whole row of nurses had started booing at the name.

Mr Hamilton looked up at the genteel nurses he'd been praising and credited with their meekness at the negotiating table. He winced slightly at this unexpected opposition from the gallery and continued with his speech. 'The number of student nurses who leave during the course of their training is well over one third and in some hospitals it is as high as four out of five …'

'That's true,' I whispered to Alex. 'A month into PTS and out of the fifty girls that started there are already five empty desks.'

'I hope you run the course; just so you don't leave Hackney, Sarah,' he said as he took my hand in his, making my heart beat distinctively faster.

'Don't you worry, I intend to stick it out to the end,' I assured him.

'Nursing is a twenty-four hours a day, seven days a week, fifty-two weeks of the year job, and this round-the-clock, round-the-year service ought to have a pay structure to reflect that uniqueness …' said Mr Hamilton.

'Hear, hear,' shouted Maddox, rising to her feet. We were all beginning to warm to this Labour politician now he was actually talking about a life we recognised as ours.

'Bloody Tories,' shouted Maddox but no one could hear her above the boos and name calling that was now taking place between the honourable members themselves. The Conservatives shook their heads and the Labour front bench nodded back vehemently as they each blamed the other for the current state of the NHS.

Now with the full attention of the House, Mr Hamilton explained the plight of the Angels of Mercy even if we did get the pay rise from the government. 'A girl who could have five O-levels, who could be qualified to go to teacher training college, is cheaper than any labourer outside an Asiatic paddy field …'

'How many O-levels did you get, Sarah?' asked Alex.

'Eight,' I replied.

He lifted his eyebrows in surprise. 'Didn't fancy teacher training college?'

'Not one bit,' I answered.

'How about a paddy field?' he asked, giving me a little nudge in my side and making me stifle a giggle.

As the evening dragged on I grew weary of the debate, as member after member added their tuppence worth. Would any of it make much difference? Were they going to put up our wages or weren't they?

'In between the cheap shots and blaming each other, are we to take it that you nurses are getting a pay rise?' asked Alex. It was approaching eleven o'clock and we were wondering how we were going to get home if the debate dragged on much longer.

'Yes, I think we are,' I replied.

'Good. Now can we get out of here?'

I nodded and took Maddox firmly by the elbow as we made our way out of Parliament and ran to the bus stop, her sign clattering along the floor as we endeavoured not to miss the last bus home.

Triumphantly Maddox and I marched into the reading room of the nurses' home where Lynch was reading a book by the fireplace, enjoying a bit of rare solitude.

'We did it. The government had to agree to increase nurses' pay,' cried Maddox, holding her banner high and punching the air. We'd been expecting a welcoming committee but the nurses' home was surprisingly quiet.

Lynch looked up from her book. A flicker of amusement flashed across her face. 'There's been a development,' she said, putting her book on the side table. 'Must have happened while you were on the bus home. You've got a new campaign to fight, Maddox, and it's against Pay As You Eat.'

'What?' asked Maddox, truly perplexed.

'They've used our minor wage increase to take away the meal allowance. We are all going to have to pay for all food and drink now; every single cup of tea will need to be budgeted for. There's going to be no more room and board, just the room.'

'But we'll be worse off than ever!' I moaned. 'I'll only be able to have a bread roll and a cup of tea for my supper.'

'Good for the waistline,' joked Lynch half-heartedly, and I gave her a weak smile back.

'Well, we just won't stand for this. I'll go to Matron first thing ...' stormed Maddox as she paced the floor working out her plan of action.

'It's out of Matron's hands. It's nationwide – one of the things Salmon and his cronies aren't dragging their heels on,' Lynch said with a wry smile.

When the changes were introduced in April 1970, a bread roll and a cup of tea was largely what sustained me for the rest of my time in the nurses' home. Things were changing; a lot of the time it was for the good, but sometimes it was for the worse – you couldn't take anything for granted any more.

12

As soon as I walked onto Geriatric Ward I knew something wasn't right. It was customary for Sister to give you the lay of the land on your first morning on a new ward, but on Geriatrics Sister Genson did not materialise out of her office. Instead, I was given instructions by Staff Nurse Clarence, a tall thin woman with piercing grey eyes and a hooked nose. She was cutting in every sense of the word; her movements were sharp like she might give you a jab in the ribs at any given moment, her eyes bore into you, her voice was high pitched and biting, and worst of all her words seemed to be dipped in acid. She eyed up her two new students with disdain. I couldn't understand Staff Nurse Clarence's hostility. She brusquely showed us round the ward without a kind word or a hint of concern for a single patient. She treated them as if they were at best minor irritants and at worst a boil that needed to be lanced – her words describing one old lady. I felt more and more uneasy but I couldn't even talk about it with my fellow student as I'd been assigned to Geriatrics with Prendergast of all people.

'I want you to make the beds up before rounds,' instructed Staff Nurse Clarence. 'And don't take any nonsense from the old girls. We have a lot of whining troublemakers on this ward who want to make every little thing into a drama – give them an inch and they'd take a mile. If we gave in to them it would be the patients running this ward. There's no room for softness here; it will get you nowhere. And as for Sister Genson, it won't be long till she joins the ranks of the patients; she's practically gaga herself,' she sneered.

Prendergast sniggered, and in her Staff Nurse Clarence recognised an ally in her war against infirmity. I was utterly shocked to see a Staff Nurse talk about a sister and the patients like she did. We students might joke about sisters from time to time but I'd never known a senior nurse be so disrespectful. I'd seen a few slapdash nurses in my time at Hackney already but Staff Nurse Clarence seemed punitive, more like a prison guard than a nurse. I hadn't felt unhappy when starting on my previous two wards, or wished I was somewhere else. It was an unwelcome and disturbing feeling, and at eighteen years of age I was at a loss to know how to tackle it.

Staff Nurse Clarence was clearly pleased at Prendergast's appreciation of her sense of humour and took her to meet some of the other nurses gathered round the nurses' desk. They were laughing, sitting on the desk and drinking cups of tea as if there wasn't a ward to run full of high-dependency patients. It was a most unfamiliar sight. I decided I'd best get on with making up the beds – nobody else seemed to be doing it. Before I'd even got started I heard the most pitiful voice of an old lady calling out weakly from the first bed at the bottom of the ward.

'Nurse,' she cried. 'Nurse, please, Nurse.'

I hurried over and glanced down at her chart to discover her name.

'What is it, Mrs Osborne?' I asked.

She looked despairingly at me with her watery eyes, her wrinkled hand grasping out for mine. As I held her hand in mine it tremored. 'What is it, Mrs Osborne?' I asked once more.

'I'm sorry, Nurse, my bed's wet. I told them last night that I needed to use the lavatory but nobody came and no one's been near me all morning. I'm wet through. Please, Nurse, help me.'

I looked at her sheets; they were soaked in urine. The smell was terrible. This poor old lady had been left since last night in wet sheets. I looked around me in horror – nobody cared. I dashed off to fetch fresh sheets and a nightdress from the linen cupboard. I looked for a screen to give Mrs Osborne some privacy but was told curtly there was only one screen on the whole ward and it was in use. I changed the sheets on Mrs Osborne's bed and she pleaded with me, 'Don't say anything, Nurse, please. I don't want them to know about my little accident. They'll say I'm not fit to look after myself, and I want to go home. I don't want to be here. My Alfred's in the next ward and we want to go home together. We don't want to be separated like this.' I was horrified and angry.

Over the next few days I witnessed more and more scenes of neglect and cruelty. Not all the staff were the same as Staff Nurse Clarence and her cronies. There were junior nurses and auxiliaries who I thought just kept their heads down and did what they could. But no one was standing up for themselves or the patients – it would have been professional suicide. For me, moving on to Geriatric Ward seemed like a Victorian nightmare after the excellent tutelage of Daddy Davis and the warmth of Infants Ward.

After three weeks on Geriatrics it was with a heavy heart that I made my way from the nurses' home across the grounds to the hospital each morning. I felt sick at the thought of spending the day there. When I was off duty I tried to push the thoughts of those horrid nurses and poor old ladies from my mind, but I couldn't – no matter how hard I studied, or when I was out with Alex, I couldn't shake off the feeling that something was wrong and I needed to do something about it – but what? I was a student nurse in her first term, Staff Nurse Clarence was a respected senior nurse; I was a nobody. And as for Sister Genson, she might have been a kindly nurse in her younger days during the war, but at sixty-five she'd already entered a premature dotage and couldn't maintain discipline on her ward or even order the supplies we desperately needed. On some wards this might have meant the staff would cut a few corners, but here under the sadistic command of Staff Nurse Clarence I'd witnessed first hand that slovenly care and bad tempered-ness had become the norm.

'Here comes Florence Nightingale,' jeered Prendergast as I came onto the ward. She had become one of Staff Nurse Clarence's clique. That morning they were gathered round a bed at the other end of the ward. Once they'd mocked me, the gang's attention returned to making fun of a distraught and confused old lady called Mrs Coker. 'I don't want to be in the workhouse. Let me out, let me out,' screamed the elderly lady. 'Please, don't let me die in the workhouse, please.'

I'd discovered that many of our older patients at Hackney remembered the time when the hospital had been a work-house. Elderly men and women came onto Geriatrics often muddled and very vulnerable, and when they saw the loom-ing Victorian building they frequently believed they were being sent to the workhouse to die. Staff Nurse Clarence and her gang did nothing to help explain that they were in hospital and needn't worry. Instead they used the threat of the workhouse to coerce patients into subordination so there was less work to do. I wanted to go to Mrs Coker but I'd tried to reassure her before, and without the backing of the rest of the nursing staff there was no hope of easing her worries, and right now I wanted to check on Mrs Osborne without drawing any unwanted attention from Staff Nurse Clarence.

There was a full porridge bowl on the table next to Mrs Osborne left untouched from breakfast, and the water jug was still completely full too. 'Didn't you fancy any breakfast this morning, Mrs Osborne?'

She looked down at her hands, embarrassed. 'I couldn't get to it, dear. And I didn't want any water in case I had another accident.'

At the thought of her starving in an NHS hospital bed I was absolutely fuming. I wanted to march over and scream at Staff Nurse Clarence, Prendergast and the rest of them, but that wouldn't help her, not in the long run, or me.

Just before Matron's morning rounds at ten o'clock, Sister Genson would pop out of her office like clockwork, ready to greet her superior at the ward door. Staff Nurse Clarence would always be at Sister's elbow, standing by to answer any tricky questions, and the patients were all too scared or confused to tell Matron about the inadequacy of their care. Sister and Staff never left Matron's side during a ward round so there was no way you could show her the true story even if you wanted to. Once the tour of the ward was finished, Sister and Staff would go to Sister's office for a debrief, leaving Matron momentarily alone. That morning as Matron was about to sweep out of Geriatrics, I was changing Miss Kilburn's soiled nightdress as discreetly as I could as the ward's one screen was already in use.

'Nurse, what do you think you are doing? Screen that bed immediately,' instructed Matron sharply.

I erupted in an explosion of anger and misery that had been building up over my last three weeks on Geriatrics. 'With what? There's only one screen,' I screamed at Matron.

'I will not tolerate impudence. Control yourself, Student Nurse Hill,' Matron said smoothly, quickly stepping towards me to take down the volume of our exchange.

'Matron, it's *sans* everything on here. There's not the basic equipment we need, and what's worse there is no care and not a scrap of compassion for the patients.'

'My office this afternoon, Nurse Hill, and bring the other student nurse with you – Prendergast, is it?' I nodded. 'We'll see if she concurs with your accusations. Three o'clock sharp,' Matron informed me before she left the ward.

Oh, God, oh God. What have I done, I thought. This was insubordination – would she send me home? Was my career over before it had even begun? There was no way Prendergast would agree with me; she was one of them. I was for the chop.

Prendergast and I stood side by side outside Matron's office waiting to be called in. It was just like being sent to the head-mistress's office, but worse; I very much wanted Matron to have a good opinion of me. My break was 2 pm to 4 pm that day, and I'd rushed back to the nurses' home to put on my best bib and tucker, a fresh pair of stockings, and to give my shoes a polish. I'd grabbed a roll and a cup of tea for my lunch, but I could barely swallow my modest meal I was so apprehensive about my interview with Matron.

'You're for the sack,' hissed Prendergast.

All morning she and the other nurses in Staff Nurse Clarence's gang had been enjoying the fate that awaited me. It was my word against theirs. Sister Genson didn't even put her head above the parapet – no one had seen her since rounds but even she must have known something was going on. I wasn't going to let Prendergast rattle me.

I told her, 'The worst they can do is send me home. They can't strike me off – I'm not even registered. Whereas your friends might never work again – have they thought of that?'

I didn't believe it myself but it was satisfying to see a look of uncertainty on Prendergast's smug round face.

At the stroke of three we heard Matron command us to enter her inner sanctum. It was just like my first morning at Hackney, as she sat neatly at her desk, piles of papers awaiting her attention, only this time she looked troubled.

'Student Nurse Hill has made a very serious accusation about certain members of the nursing team on Geriatric Ward,' began Matron.

'I've never seen anything untoward, Matron,' interrupted Prendergast.

Matron fixed her with a look that penetrated even Prendergast's thick skin. Reprimanded, the student nurse now remembered her place and looked silently at her hands while Matron continued uninterrupted.

'I do not like tittle-tattle. I will not tolerate insubordination. But when an allegation is made about the quality of care given to patients in this hospital I take that most seriously. Nurse Hill, what can a girl only at the very beginning of her nurse training be thinking to challenge her senior colleagues? What do you hope to gain?'

'Nothing, Matron. I just want them to be kind to the old ladies. I don't want to see patients frightened, or hungry, or in unnecessary pain. I just want us to do our best for them. To give them the care we'd want ourselves,' I burst out. 'It's so unfair, Matron. I hadn't planned on telling you like that, I just couldn't help it.'

Matron appeared to be unmoved. She simply asked me to list when I thought the care given was insufficient; I obediently and silently wrote it down. In turn she asked Prendergast whether she agreed with each claim. Prendergast gave an unwavering denial of every count. Matron shook her head and sighed and then we were dismissed. I think both Prendergast and I returned to the ward with heavy hearts that afternoon. No one asked us about the interview even though it must have been the talk of the whole ward. Everyone just got on with their work quietly, even Staff Nurse Clarence, and Sister Genson remained in her office as always.

The journey to Geriatric Ward the next afternoon felt longer than ever. My legs were heavy, my eyes and head hurt from a sleepless night. Even the very air felt oppressive as I trudged to work. It looked like rain, and dark clouds were forming over the hospital. I was sure it would thunder. This is going to be my last day in Hackney, I thought. By this evening I will be on the train heading back to my parents' house, leaving behind my friends, my home, my career and Alex. The previous evening I'd wept down the phone in the corridor of the nurses' home while I told my boyfriend the whole sorry tale. Not big heavy sobs, but soundlessly, with my face turned to the wall so no one would see, while I'd listened to Alex telling me everything would be all right. 'I'd do anything for you, Sarah,' he comforted. How I now clung to those words; I wanted to wrap them round to buffer me from my impending doom.

When I reached Geriatrics I made an effort to compose myself. I must face up to those sneering faces. I didn't want them to see they'd got the better of me. No doubt Staff Nurse Clarence had already been instructed to give me my marching orders. I pushed through the doors but was taken aback – had I stepped onto the wrong ward? There were a few familiar faces but a lot of new ones too, busily hurrying up and down the ward changing beds, helping the patients eat, laughing, brushing hair and reading letters. A hive of caring activity appeared to be taking place at every bedside. I felt like I'd walked into a dream.

Slightly shaky, I made my way towards the nurses' desk in the middle of the long ward. There sat a staff nurse I did not know.

'Ah, you must be Student Nurse Hill,' she said. 'I'm Foley. Pleased to meet you. Would you please see if Mrs Osborne would like a bath today?'

'Where's Staff Nurse Clarence?' I asked, a little dumbfounded.

'Haven't you heard? I thought *you* would have been the first to know.'

I shook my head.

'Sister Genson's decided to retire, bless her. So Matron's reorganised the staff, moved a few of the old faces to new wards – shaken them up a bit.'

I stared at Staff Nurse Foley in wonder at first and then I realised what Matron had done. I started grinning like the Cheshire cat.

'Oh, and Hill. When you've given Mrs Osborne her bath we've a lot of new equipment arriving this afternoon. I want you to take delivery and check we've got everything we need. Chop, chop,' instructed our efficient new Staff Nurse as she returned to writing up the reports from night duty. Then she looked up and called me back. 'Hill, message from Matron. Lower your skirt. Miniskirts are not appropriate for student nurses or any nurse in this hospital. That'll be all for now.'

'Yes, Staff,' I said as I attempted to pull my skirt down a little. All my friends had shortened their uniforms. Trust Matron not to miss that, I smiled. Good old Matron. I wasn't going to lower my skirt, though.

My shift flew by. It was my first truly happy day in weeks. Mrs Osborne looked transformed after a bath and a hair wash. I set her hair in rollers and helped her find her make-up. Before long she was looking at herself in a tortoiseshell hand mirror she'd brought with her in a red leather vanity case. She smeared a little pale pink lipstick on her mouth and gave a satisfied smile. Her hair was now in splendid shiny slivery-grey curls and neatly piled on top of her head. She wore a pale silk lavender nightdress and bed jacket with ivory lace at the neck and cuffs. She'd brought all these things with her but no one had unpacked them. She'd been too frightened to wear the nightdress for fear of spoiling it, but now she looked resplendent in her bed, sitting up and resting on a stack of freshly laundered pillows.

'I wore this nightdress on my honeymoon,' she whispered. 'We went to Bangor.'

'It's beautiful,' I said admiringly.

'Still fits like a glove. I expect that's due to not having had children and all the dancing and prancing about on stage,' she said wistfully.

I could see for the first time the woman she truly was – not a frail little old lady who couldn't care for herself, but a vibrant actress who'd entertained and held the attention of theatres full of people for decades. A loving wife who was missing her husband. She rummaged round in her vanity case and brought out a beautiful turquoise and sea-green art deco compact. She opened it and dabbed powder onto her face.

'Always wear a little powder if you can, dear,' she told me as she inspected her face in the mirror. 'My mother always used to say to me, "Daisy, always look respectable, you never know who you might bump into,"' she explained, closing the compact once more with a satisfying click.

'You look lovely, Mrs Osborne,' I told her.

'Thank you, dear. I feel much, much better. It's amazing what a hot meal, a bath and a bit of lipstick can do for a woman,' she told me. 'You don't have to be a beauty but every woman can look attractive no matter how old if she just makes the most of herself. I hope my Alfred's got a nice young nurse like you looking after him. Mind, I wouldn't want her skirts to be as short as yours, set the old boy's ticker right off!' she cackled, giving me a nudge in the ribs.

'Would you like me to pop over to the men's ward and see how Mr Osborne is doing?'

'Yes, please,' she said, breaking out into a smile at the thought of her Alfred. 'We haven't been separated for over sixty years. We toured together – never had a night apart. We sang, you know, in the musical halls. We even sang for a duke once – I can't remember which one now, but I know he was a duke.'

I practically skipped out of the ward and across to the Male Geriatric Ward where I spotted Lynch changing the bandages on a patient's foot.

'Hill, what are you doing over here?' Lynch called to me in surprise.

'Looking for Mr Osborne. His wife's on my ward.'

'He's a card. Bed on the left near the window. Watch yourself, he's a bit of a pincher,' she told me, biting her lower lip so she wouldn't laugh.

I found Mr Osborne not in bed but sitting in a chair next to the window reading a copy of *Variety*. He was wearing a brown and black striped dressing gown tied with a red cord and red velvet slippers to match. His hair, though grey, was still thick and wavy and he had twinkly blue eyes. Yes, I thought, he and Mrs Osborne must have been quite a pair. Lynch bustled over, never one to miss out on any gossip, and we agreed Mr Osborne should come to have tea on my ward at four o'clock as a surprise for his wife.

Just before it was time for tea, Staff Nurse Foley and I started to set up a little cluster of tables and chairs at the far end of the ward and laid out the tea things. We even managed to rustle up some cake and nice biscuits. The old ladies watched us curiously while all the nursing staff helped them into robes and slippers so the ones who could get out of bed joined our little café, and the ones who couldn't were propped up on pillows with their tea things on a tray.

At the stroke of four, in strode Mr Osborne. He was followed by Lynch, who was pushing an upright piano with the assistance of one of the hospital porters. The ward lit up with surprised and delighted faces. A fair few of the other old gentleman from the opposite ward came across to enjoy our tea party, accompanied by a few of my fellow student nurses, including Daniels who was pushing an old gentleman in a wheelchair with his foot in a cast. We waved excitedly at each other: this wasn't on the curriculum for nurse training. Mr Osborne, with the confident air of a seasoned performer, went to his wife's bedside and offered her his hand.

'Alfred, what's all this?' she asked in delight.

'Nurse,' instructed Mr Osborne as previously arranged. I scurried over to the upright piano and began to play. Finally the fruitless hours of my musical education were paying off as Mr Osborne broke into 'Daisy, Daisy'. He helped his wife out of bed and together they strolled arm in arm to the piano. They led the other patients in a chorus of 'My Old Man Said Follow the Van' and 'There Was I, Waiting at the Church'.

Lynch whispered to me, 'I wouldn't expect a nice young lady like you to know how to play musical-hall tunes.'

'My grandfather used to sing them to us on Sundays,' I whispered back. 'After church.'

I saw Matron's head through the glass window in the ward doors. She wouldn't come in – she couldn't officially approve of this sort of carry-on – but I swear I saw her smile for the first time since I came to Hackney.

13

I hovered in the doorway of the reading room. Alex looked worried. Awkwardly perched on a chintz armchair, he was listening to Wade telling him all about her first assisted delivery of twins in every intricate detail. I should have rushed in and rescued him immediately, but it was so sweet. I watched him following Wade's gory tale in silent horror, too polite and too reserved to ask her to stop as she used a cushion to elaborately illustrate her point.

In the background was the giant black and white television set. As a few student nurses gathered round and turned up the volume, watching a large spinning crown, I realised the 1970 Miss World Competition was about to start. It was being hosted at the Royal Albert Hall and Maddox had been going on and on about what a disgrace it was all week, especially when it was announced that South Africa was sending two entrants, one white and one black. Actually, I was pretty disgusted by that myself, but I didn't see why Maddox thought the competition was the end of the world – I just accepted it as a bit of fun, something you could watch with your granny even. I drifted towards the television set as a montage of girls and flags flittered across the screen. Alex saw me and rushed over, eager to be away from Wade.

'Happy Birthday, Sarah,' he whispered in my ear as I leant against him.

We watched the camera pan across the wide expanse of the grand hall and settle momentarily on the glittering stage of neatly fitted hexagons. Steps led up to a semi-circular podium decorated with large Grecian columns, all enshrined by a shimmering curtain. A panel of judges grinned at the camera as Michael Aspel introduced them one by one. I didn't recognise any of them immediately except Joan Collins, who shimmied her shoulders and batted her eyelashes for the camera in a plunging V-neck gown with tiny shoulder straps, her hair a mass of lush dark curls scooped up high on her head.

I looked down at my own dress for the evening, a white and light green floral number with a high-necked white collar and cuffs, teamed with black shoes, handbag and coat. My hair was down like always when I was off duty, so long now it reached my elbows – I was in desperate need of a haircut. My ensemble was the smartest thing in my wardrobe although not exactly evening wear. I wasn't like the elegant Miss Collins in her long dangly earrings and exposed cleavage, but then Alex wasn't in black tie either. He'd donned a brown suit for the occasion, and I'd never seen him in a suit before so I knew he was making an effort. I was a bit worried about how much this birthday meal was going to cost him; he'd insisted we go to the Post Office Tower to celebrate on my night off. I'd offer to pay for myself of course but I knew he wouldn't accept it, not tonight.

'Did you see there was a bomb exploded under a BBC outside broadcast van there tonight?' Alex asked me.

'At the Albert Hall? No. Why?' I responded, shocked out of my reverie on the girls' national costumes.

'The Angry Brigade,' said Alex.

'What have those layabouts got to be angry about?' chimed in Wade.

'I think it's about Vietnam,' I said softly.

'What's Vietnam got to do with us?' she shrieked.

I thought of my best friend Sue and the people in the street who'd spat at her and shouted comments about slitty eyes, and hugged myself as we watched Bob Hope wander across the stage. He was going badly off script.

'I'm very, very happy to be here at this cattle market tonight – I've been backstage checking the calves,' joked the American comedian.

'God, I bet his gag writer didn't do that one,' said Alex.

'I'd hate you to think I was a dirty old man because I never give women a second thought. My first thought covers everything,' he waffled. There was about the same level of laughter in the huge Albert Hall as there was in our modest reading room – very little.

Suddenly we heard rattles coming from somewhere in the audience. Bob Hope's eyes darted about, looking confused and then worried. Another rattle sounded, and then another and then another until you couldn't hear a word he was saying. Something white exploded onto the stage and then what looked like vegetables were being thrown at him. The camera showed the audience and suddenly a woman stood up with a sign and shouted her message: 'We're not beautiful, we're not ugly, we're angry.' Woman after woman stood shouting and booing as Bob Hope ran off the stage. Then we all gasped in surprise as a woman stood and threw a shoe onto the stage and shouted out her slogan, 'Miss Fortune demands equal pay for women.' She blinked into the spotlights that were shining on her, her fringe in her eyes, in a scruffy jumper and jeans.

'Oh my. It's Maddox,' I gasped.

'Blimey, if I'd known I'd have lent her an old pair of stilettos. Those boring old pumps don't make much of an impact,' said Wade.

We watched as security men made their way into the audience and removed the women, who kicked and screamed as they were dragged away.

The camera quickly returned to Bob Hope, who was back on stage saying, 'This is a nice conditioning course to Vietnam,' to an explosion of relieved laughter from the previously meek audience.

We all stood willing the camera to go back to the audience to find out what had happened to Maddox, but it didn't.

'What should we do?' I asked Alex.

'I don't know what we can do.'

'We can't go for dinner now. Something might have happened to her.'

'Hill,' said Wade sharply. 'What can you do? Nothing. Don't let Maddox's goody two-shoes shenanigans spoil your birthday. Now off for dinner, you two, you'll miss your table.'

Alex and I looked at each other and remained rooted to the spot. I wanted to go for our lovely dinner, I wanted to pretend we hadn't seen anything, but it felt wrong to just go. Then the decision was taken out of our hands.

Daniels rushed in. 'Hill, pay phone for you. It's Maddox. She sounds like she's had a terrible fright.'

I looked at Alex and Wade. We were all thinking the same thing – what has that girl got herself into?

Alex and I huddled together for warmth, our breath mingled in the frosty November air as we conspicuously peered through the railings opposite the Albert Memorial. There was still a few bobbies patrolling Kensington Gore on this eventful evening, and the last thing we wanted to do was draw attention to ourselves and get arrested as would-be protestors.

'Maddox, Maddox!' I half-shouted in a stage whisper.

The figure of Prince Albert under the huge canopy starred down at us in all his gothic magnificence and made me feel uneasy. The park looked like it went on forever in the dark, shadowy tree after shadowy tree creating an impenetrable fortress – we were too timid to venture beyond the railings.

'How far do you think she went in?' asked Alex.

'I don't know.'

'You'd be lost in there till the sun comes up if you lost sight of the road. Without a light you'd lose your bearings very quickly.'

Maddox had been hiding in a phone box when she'd rung to request we come and get her, but the sight of her fellow protestors being manhandled into police riot vans during the call had made her jumpy. She'd said she was going to hide in Kensington Gardens until we came for her, and then hung up.

I was just about to call her again when a policeman started sauntering towards us.

'Quick,' said Alex, spinning me around to face him and then kissing me against the railings until the policeman passed us by.

I felt exhilarated and a little dizzy. I started to call Maddox's name gently again, and was wondering how much longer we could do this for, when a small figure stuck their head out from behind the memorial.

'Maddox,' I hissed. 'Come here right now. The coast is clear.'

Maddox starting doing a half-run half-tiptoe down the steps. I heard Alex snicker under his breath when we realised she was only wearing one shoe. We then pulled her over the railings and she fell into my arms. Alex didn't waste a second. He hailed a passing hackney carriage and we bungled Maddox into the taxi. As we sped away from the Royal

Albert Hall, into the park and over the Serpentine, we all heaved a collective sigh of relief. Once the bright lights of Marble Arch were in view, quiet, uptight Maddox threw her head back and began to laugh, her shoulders shaking, her hands holding her belly until she slumped back spent onto the back seat of the cab. As the grand department store windows on Oxford Street flashed by she began to talk rapidly, barely drawing breath about her adventures that evening.

'I didn't get off duty in time to meet everyone before they went in. I missed the protest outside the hall completely, so I just had to go in on my own. I was sitting there and there were all these nice people around me, the sort of people we see every day in Hackney – there for a bit of so-called family entertainment – and it made me feel bad about the whole thing. I was just about to leave and forget it all when Bob Hope started making jokes about it being a cattle market and saying he'd been backstage to check the calves, ha ha ha. And I felt so angry and then I heard those football rattles go off. I looked up and there were all these leaflets falling down like confetti and flour being thrown and I thought I need to do something. But I realised I didn't bring anything; I'd been in such a rush. I had sneaked some old vegetables from the kitchen to throw but I'd forgotten them and I don't know what came over me, I took off one of my shoes and I threw it onto the stage!' Maddox beamed with pride at her own ingenuity.

'We know, we saw it on the TV,' I told her.

'I realised if Matron found out I'd been out on my ear. That's when I ran,' explained Maddox.

The taxi was racing through Marylebone and I saw the Post Office Tower come into view, like a spacecraft or a huge beacon reaching towards the sky, dwarfing the blocks of offices that stood in its shadow.

'Stop here, please, driver,' instructed Alex. He pulled out his wallet and gave a few notes to Maddox. 'This will get you back to Hackney. Now, we're going to see if we can still get a table for Sarah's birthday,' he said very firmly as he took my hand and opened the door of the cab.

'Oh, yes,' said Maddox a little bashfully. 'Have a lovely meal!' she called as Alex shut the door of the taxi and tapped on the roof. I heaved a long sigh as the taxi pulled away with Maddox waving through the back window.

Alex and I stood behind a couple in the lift. As we went up, up, up, I started to feel dizzy from the overwhelming smell of the lady's musky perfume. They seemed larger than life standing in front of us, her in a huge floor-length mink coat and him in an expensive-looking long woollen winter coat and hat – proper grown-ups. Alex and I silently held hands, our backs pressed to the lift wall, until finally the doors opened and the glamorous couple stepped out confidently ahead of us and disappeared into the throng at The Top of the Tower. We crept forwards in the direction of the receptionist, who sat at a red leather upholstered desk against a backdrop of royal blue walls. Two white telephones posi-

tioned in front of her were ringing, but she was busy looking through papers – checking off who'd missed their tables,
no doubt. A large red clock above her head was telling us
we'd missed our reservation. We nervously approached the
desk – her red hair was neatly arranged on top of her head,
she had bright red nails and lipstick, but her eye shadow and
dress were deep blue. I wondered if she'd been instructed to
match the colour scheme of the reception or whether it was
just coincidence. She looked up and smiled.

'We had a reservation for eight o'clock,' began Alex
timidly. 'But I'm afraid we had an emergency and we are a
little late,' he explained, glancing up at the clock – it was
almost nine.

'Take a seat,' instructed the receptionist, pointing to a
curved red leather bench in the corner. We obediently sat
and kept our eyes fixed on the large floral arrangement that
took up the entire coffee table in front of us. The receptionist picked up the receiver of one of the white telephones and
made a call but we couldn't hear what she was saying. It was
going to be so embarrassing if they turned us away, and I
knew Alex would take it very badly even though it wasn't his
fault in the least. We waited for what felt forever to be
dismissed but it wasn't really much more than five minutes.
Eventually, the *maître d'* came bustling over to us, the coat
tails of his penguin suit flapping behind him.

'Ah, bonsoir Mademoiselle, Monsieur. I believe it is
Mademoiselle's birthday?' We nodded. 'We have kept a very
special table just for you. Come this way,' he said with a

dramatic sweep of his hand. Stunned, we followed him to our table.

Alex and I grinned at each other over the tops of our blue and white menus. We had a cosy table with two dark blue leather chairs and a view from the spinning tower looking out all over London. Long windows lined the circular dining room in a perfect circle – it felt so free, so exciting, like being in another world. It was amazing to see the city twinkling, with its ever-changing pattern of lights telling a million different stories just for us. Glancing around the restaurant, there was an outer ring of diners by the windows and an inner circle orbiting what looked like a giant red cake stand covered in dishes – a roast chicken, and all manner of *hors d'oeuvres* and *crudités*. A waiter was busy pushing a trolley serving coffee and desserts round and round the middle of the two circles. I looked back at my menu. There were no prices for anything except to say there was a minimum charge of £2.50 and a cover charge of 40p. That meant it was going to be expensive. I decided we'd skip the fiddly bits and go straight to the main course, and tried to work out what would be the most inexpensive dish. Would *Le Filet Grillé* cost less than *Les Scampi et Frites*? Oh, and they had asparagus, I'd loved that ever since I'd had it on the plane flying to boarding school from Scotland when I was ten, but I would forgo it, and go for *petit pois* instead – it was the wrong time of year for asparagus anyway. I looked up, ready to ask Alex what he was having, but he was studying the menu with a look of panic on his face. Oh no, he really couldn't afford this – I wondered if we could just leave.

He whispered to me, 'Sarah, it's all in French.'

'Yes?' I replied, not understanding why this should cause him such alarm.

'Do you speak French?'

'Yes,' I answered, pushing down the urge to reply *mais oui.*

'Good. Order me the chicken.'

'Alex, you always have the chicken.'

'Chicken never lets you down.'

I shook my head and let out a sigh of relief. We laughed and I ordered him the chicken. It felt like we were on top of the world.

14

I tapped my fingers on the shiny silver buckle fastened to my new blue belt as I considered what to serve each patient for their dinner. I was now in my second year as a student, and that January night I really felt I'd gone up a notch as I was the most senior nurse on duty in the Male Medical Ward. It fell to me to serve the dinners to the patients from the hot trolley – deciding on the dishes and portion sizes appropriate for each man. Only a few weeks into yet another new ward, I could now easily smooth over Mr Gill as he complained about being given soup and rice pudding *again* while eyeing up the remaining dish on my trolley. It was braised steak, carrots and mashed potato destined for Mr Cassidy in a side ward.

I paused with my trolley outside old man Cassidy's room and thought about Alex. I wasn't due to start my shift until ten o'clock that evening but had been called in at six as Staff Nurse was off sick and I'd no option but to break another date. This was my ninth night shift in a row and I had barely seen my boyfriend for a month. Sister Steadman assured me that I only had to do tomorrow night and then I could have a day off and move back onto days. I really hoped so; I'd had so little sleep and it was playing havoc with my love life. I'd promised Alex faithfully on the phone that I'd see him tomorrow for a couple of hours before I went back on night duty; I prayed Sister wouldn't make me break my promise.

I was roused from my thoughts of life off the ward by the sound of Mr Cassidy half coughing and half shouting at the houseman in his room.

'What does a veritable duckling like you know? I want to see Dr Holmes,' rasped Mr Cassidy.

'Now, now, Mr Cassidy. It doesn't pay to get over-excited. I've sent off for the results on your chest X-ray and sputum …'

'My what?'

'Spit,' explained Dr Guy Fleming, taking his stethoscope from around his neck. 'I'll listen once more to your chest but all you can do is rest in this room and remain in isolation.'

'Nonsense. It's my boy Charlie; he wants me out of the way. How much is he paying you to keep me in here?'

Dr Guy laughed nervously and continued to examine the old man, his long back arched high as he bent over this small but stout East End villain.

'We're very concerned about your breathing. Your lungs are struggling at the moment – we need to get them in order again,' said Dr Guy gently.

In between Dr Holmes the consultant and Sister Steadman the departmental sister, Dr Guy was having a rough time of it at the moment.

'I'm on call so if you have any problems breathing just alert the nurse and I'll be here like a shot,' finished Dr Guy as he bid Mr Cassidy a hasty farewell and departed the side ward. Wrapping his stethoscope back around his neck and running a hand through his tousled brown hair, he looked exhausted. His eyes were wearily narrowing behind his round spectacles. My humble opinion was Dr Guy needed a hot meal and a sleep more than Mr Cassidy.

'Ah, Nurse Hill,' said the young doctor quietly as he spotted me waiting with my trolley. 'I suspect Mr Cassidy has TB. He needs to remain in isolation to prevent spreading the disease with all that coughing. I'll know more tomorrow when the results come back.'

I smiled and nodded as Dr Guy dashed off to try and get some shut-eye in the doctors' sitting room before he was called back again. As usual he was dressed in his boarding school pyjamas underneath his white coat. They were too short in the leg; he must have had them since he was twelve. He was one of the nice housemen, well-to-do like most of them, but kind and concerned, and he knew what he was doing, which was pretty rare.

Once it got to eleven o'clock and most of the patients were asleep I went into Sister's office to write up the evening observations and prepare the charts for the next day. I thought back to earlier that week and chuckled to myself. Lynch had been on Male Medical too and we'd been making beds. Suddenly, I heard her call my name from the other end of the ward.

'Hill, are you still stripping?' shouted Lynch at the top of her lungs. Peals of laughter had broken out from every bed, as I stood there red faced, and Lynch had a puzzled look on her face. She hurried down to my end of the ward. 'I don't see what's so funny,' she'd said, a little bemused.

Now, through the window I watched Simon Reed, a heroin addict that Gerald, Maddox's boyfriend, had found in the churchyard at St Barnabas. He was the first heroin addict I'd seen. He paced up and down, unable to sleep. The dark green dressing gown with a thick black cord we'd acquired for him flapped about his scrawny limbs. His black wavy shoulder-length hair, sunken brown eyes and pale face made him a haunting figure on the dimly lit ward. During the day he was fitful and erratic; lucid and surprisingly thoughtful one minute and then rambling and increasingly hostile the next. We'd attempted to contact his next of kin, but his only relative was a younger sister, a student nurse herself at another London hospital. She said she'd try and come in but we hadn't seen her, and in any case I didn't think Simon would even know her as he frequently mistook any blonde nurse for his sibling.

He rapped at the door. I wearily got up and answered it. I'd had a long week of his non-stop chatter and demands for coffee and cornflakes all night long – I didn't expect tonight to be any different.

'Who's that old codger who's got a room to himself?' Simon said. 'Why's he so special?'

'Mr Cassidy is in isolation,' I explained.

'Cassidy. Charlie Cassidy's old man?' he asked.

I shuddered a little at the memory of the Cassidy brothers on Infants Ward but I didn't answer his question; instead I asked my own. 'Do you want coffee and cornflakes?'

Simon sat down uninvited on Sister's desk and began coughing. For a man in his twenties he had the breathing capacity of an eighty-year-old, not that he let that hold him back when he was riled. Lynch had told me that only yesterday he'd thrown a water jug at Sister while she'd been encouraging him to get some air and have a little walk in the hospital grounds. The jug had missed her temple by an inch and landed at the feet of Dr Holmes, dampening his highly polished brogues and elegantly tailored trousers. Sherlock (as we called him behind his back) had referred him to a psychiatric consultant but he hadn't been in yet to make an assessment.

'How come Cassidy's allowed visitors at this time of night?' Simon demanded.

'He's not.'

'You want your eyes testing, Nurse, because I've seen at least four blokes go into his room in the last half hour.'

'Back to your bed, Mr Reed,' I instructed as I hastened off to investigate.

I should have known better by now and done my paperwork at the nurses' desk on the ward to keep a better eye on the likes of Mr Cassidy. When I approached his room I heard the usual coughing and there was a light shining from underneath his door, so he was up. I peeped in through the window and saw Mr Cassidy sitting up in bed, a cigar on the go, a glass of whisky in front of him, cards in his hands, surrounded by four disreputable-looking members of his gang. He'd set up a poker school during my shift. Oh, help. Sister was going to have my guts for garters if she found out.

I heard one of his henchmen say, 'We've been to see what Charlie's up to. By the looks of it he's not doing anything he shouldn't – well, not where the business is concerned anyway. He's with a bit of skirt tonight. Some nurse who he's amusing himself with while his missus is in the family way again.'

'Watch him. I want to know every move that boy makes while I'm in here. If he tries to pull the wool over my eyes I want to know about it.'

I'd heard enough of their sordid intrigues. Furious at Cassidy, and at myself for letting him get one over on me, I flung open the door, but got very little reaction. Not one of them looked up. They just continued with their game.

'Mr Cassidy, visiting hours are long over and you're supposed to be in isolation. Alcohol and gambling are strictly off limits too,' I scolded.

'Don't get your knickers in a twist, Nurse,' he condescended. 'We're just doing a little bit of business. If Mohammed can't go to the mountain and all that,' he scoffed and then wheezed his guts up.

'Hackney Hospital is not a mountain and you most definitely are not a prophet. All of you get out,' I said firmly, pointing my finger in the direction of the exit.

Not one of them budged an inch. They all looked to Old Man Cassidy.

'I never could say no to a lady. We'll call it a night, boys. I'll see you tomorrow,' sneered the reprobate. 'And don't forget – I want a full report.'

They each threw their hand down and sauntered past me, smiling and looking me up and down. I stood my ground and waited until the last of the scoundrels had departed and switched off the light.

'Good night, Mr Cassidy,' I said, trying to keep the resentment out of my voice.

After all that I needed a strong cup of tea. We weren't allowed to drink on the wards but I'd been there for hours and needed a break. I installed myself at the nurses' desk in the middle of the long ward and kept my eyes firmly fixed on the ward doors should any of Mr Cassidy's out-of-hours visitors return. I cradled the cup and saucer and took the tiniest sip when I saw a silhouette I knew all too well appear at the top of the ward. Instantly I dropped the full cup of tea, saucer and all, into the waste-paper basket at my feet. Matron was making a surprise inspection – this just wasn't my night.

To my relief every man was in his bed and Matron made her tour with me without incident.

'All in order, Nurse Hill,' she told me as she left.

'Goodnight, Matron,' I replied with a sigh of relief.

'You can take your tea out of the bin now,' she added, before disappearing into the night.

How did she know? And if tea was outlawed, imagine what she'd have made of poker, black-market liquor and cigars.

15

It was just after six o'clock in the evening but the sky was so dark on that wintry January night it could have been the middle of the night. The rain was rattling against the window of my small bedroom in the nurses' home as I brushed out my hair. I was smartening myself up a bit before going down to see Alex. I'd only been up an hour. When I'd come off night duty I'd gone to the nurses' dining room to get something to eat with the other girls – breakfast for them but supper for me – but instead of getting straight off to bed as soon as I'd finished I sat gossiping until it was past ten o'clock. It was such a miserable day, Alex and I were just going to cosy up on the sofa and watch *Monty Python* in the nurses' home instead of going over to his maisonette like we usually did.

I tucked my feet under me and rested my head in Alex's lap, and we laughed together at our favourite show. He gently smoothed out my hair with his hands and I felt myself relax and wonder what life would be like, just the two of us in a little cottage in the middle of nowhere. That was Alex's dream but I wasn't sure if it was mine.

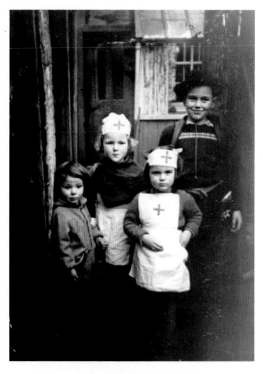

Left: Sarah, aged three, showing early signs of her nursing vocation! With siblings Bridget (left), Jane (second from left) and William (right).

Below left: Sarah's father Eric (second from left) meets Queen Elizabeth II at the opening of the Ben Cruachan Dam, 15 October 1965.

Below right: Sarah's mother Margaret napping in the car.

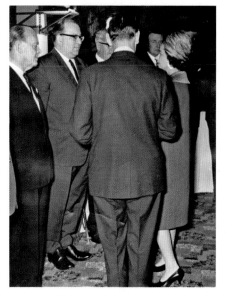

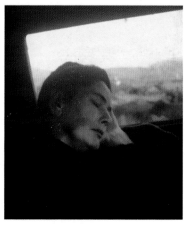

Right: Sarah babysitting a neighbour's children in Scotland, 1966.

Below left: Sarah walks along the shoreline in Wales, just before leaving for nurse training in 1969.

Below right: Sarah's father Eric tends the strawberry beds in the family's walled garden, Wales, 1969.

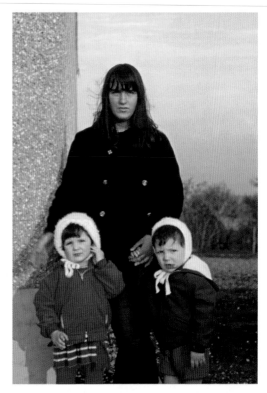

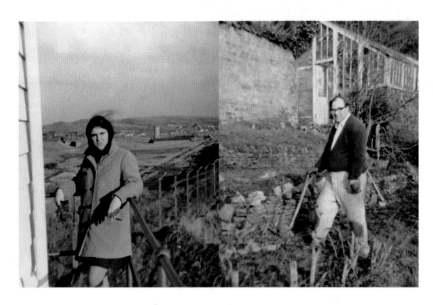

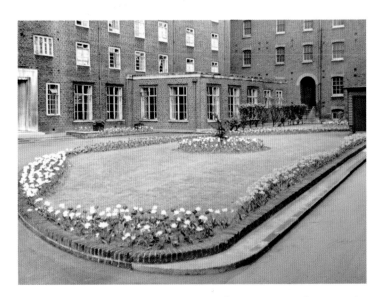

Above: The main entrance to Hackney Hospital Nurses' Home – Sarah's first view of her new home.

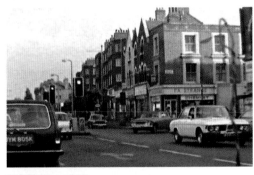

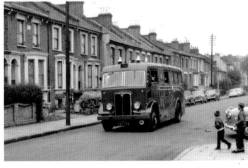

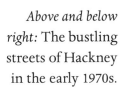

Above and below right: The bustling streets of Hackney in the early 1970s.

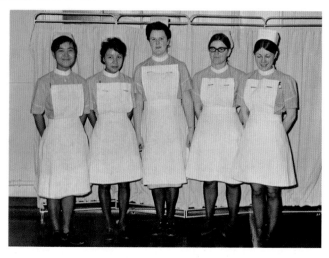

Above: Sarah (second from right), eager to get started, lines up with her student nurse classmates in their spotless new uniforms for Preliminary Training School photographs, January 1970.

Below left: Sarah's training syllabus and her newly purchased nurse's watch, both of which she treasures to this day.

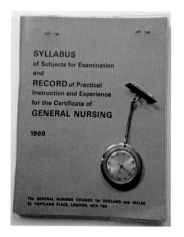

SYLLABUS
of Subjects for Examination
and
RECORD of Practical
Instruction and Experience
for the Certificate of
GENERAL NURSING

1969

The GENERAL NURSING COUNCIL for ENGLAND and WALES
23, PORTLAND PLACE, LONDON, W1A 1BA

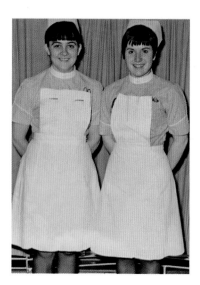

Above: Lynch (right) poses for her Preliminary Training School photograph in 1969.

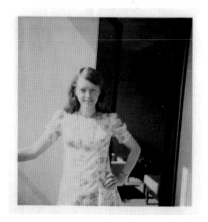

Above left: Appleton all dressed up for a night out.

Below right: Sarah (with a too-short skirt) and Appleton (right) at the Infants' Ward Christmas party, 1971.

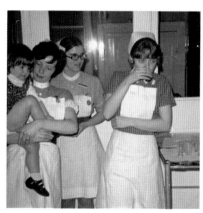

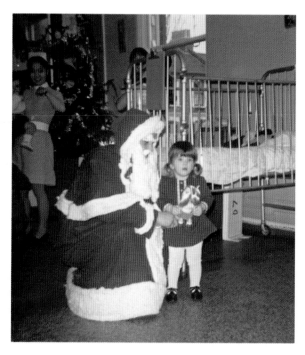

Left: Father Christmas makes a special visit to Infants' Ward, December 1971.

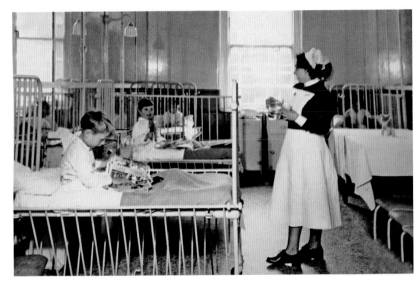

Above: A sister attending to her charges on Children's Ward.

Below left: Sarah happy to be back on Infants' Ward again with two cheeky little patients. *Below right:* Sarah returns to the family house in Wales for a holiday, summer 1971.

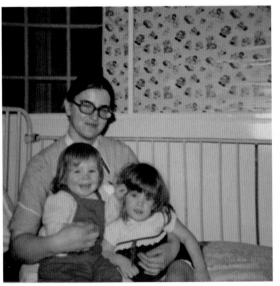

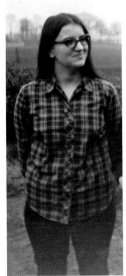

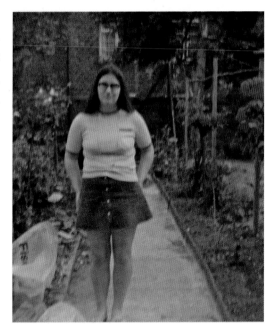

Right: Sarah shows off another too-short skirt in the garden of the girls' flat on Balls Pond Road, summer 1972.

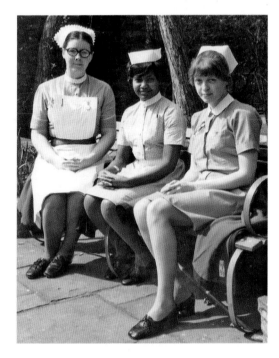

Left: Appleton (right) takes a well-earned break with colleagues in the hospital gardens, 1973.

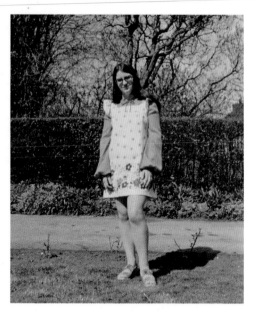

Above: Sarah proudly shows off her new-look bell sleeves and linen dress, bought in London's West End, summer 1973.

Below: Many years later, Sarah receives her MBE from Queen Elizabeth II for services to children and families. Buckingham Palace, February 2006.

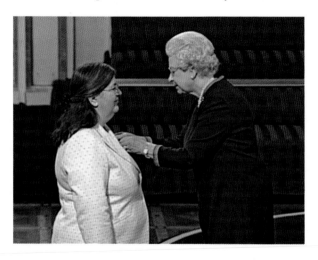

Suddenly we heard a blood-curdling scream just outside the window of the sitting room. I sat bolt upright and trembled all over. I was used to all manner of shouting, screaming and cursing by now, but that was a sound of terror I'd never heard before – something was very, very wrong.

'I'm going to check outside,' said Alex calmly. I rose to go with him. 'No, Sarah. Wait here.'

I nodded and Alex left. I strained to hear something but everything had gone deadly silent except for the ticking of the clock on the little stone mantelpiece. Time seemed to be moving very slowly. I was afraid, very afraid.

Then I heard Alex call my name. I jumped up and ran out barefoot into the howling rain and I found him crouched on the lawn next to a girl in a nurses' cloak like mine. She was utterly still, lying face down in a shallow, dirty puddle, her blonde curls spread out around her, bobbing on the scummy surface of the water.

I knelt down next to Alex. 'Go and telephone the hospital for help,' I told him as he immediately jumped into action.

I took a deep breath and rolled the girl onto her back and checked her airways. She was unconscious but still breathing, thank God. I placed her carefully into the recovery position on her side. I was taken aback to see a thick red ring round her throat and next to her in the puddle was a piece of black cord from a dressing gown.

*   *   *

I'd left the nurses' home just before ten o'clock but I'd felt ill at ease in my nurse's cloak. Normally it was such a comfort – I was so proud to wear it, with its scarlet lining, but tonight I could barely bring myself to put on my uniform. Alex was still being interviewed by the police in Home Sister's sitting room and I didn't even get the chance to say goodnight. I'd already told the police all I knew, after the team from the hospital had rushed down to claim one of our own. It had been Maddox who recognised the half-strangled girl – she was a first-year student from Ireland called Alice Murray. I didn't know her very well, but I'd seen her about, jiving with the other Irish girls to Elvis records on a Dansette in the hallway, using the doorknob as a dance partner. Alice was only eighteen, pretty and always up for a good time. There'd been rumours she was having a fling with a local – a married man.

I was surprised to see Sister and Dr Holmes still on duty as I arrived on the ward. They were in deep discussion with one of the police officers who'd interviewed me earlier. It appeared that Sister and Sherlock were being subjected to the same lacklustre cross-examination by Detective Constable Bulmer, who was making notes in a small black notebook with a stubby pencil. I could see just about every patient straining to hear what was being said. Surely they should be talking in Sister's office – what was going on? Sister saw me and called me over.

'Nurse Hill, Mr Reed and Mr Cassidy are both missing. Do you know anything that could help us discover where they might be?'

'I don't know,' I responded, more than a little taken aback by this turn of events.

'Oh, it's you again,' said the policeman suspiciously.

Sister glared at Detective Bulmer. 'Nurse Hill, is there anything you might have heard that could tell us where they are?' she asked me again.

'Mr Cassidy was worried about his son,' I told her. 'Worried he'd do some deals behind his back, but by the sounds of it Charlie Cassidy's more interested in chasing women than taking over his father's empire.'

'You know Charlie Cassidy?' sneered the detective.

'Detective Constable, this is a hospital,' snapped Sister. 'We know every Cassidy man, woman and child. If that is a crime you may as well arrest the majority of Hackney's staff.'

'And why was Mr Cassidy staying in a side ward?' asked the detective of Dr Holmes, turning his back on me and Sister Steadman.

Sister replied for doctor. 'The man has TB.'

The policeman ignored her but scribbled TB in his notebook and continued to ask his questions of Dr Holmes. 'And what about Mr Reed?'

I started to answer, 'Mr Reed was erratic. You know that yourself, Sister. He was having problems breathing ...'

'That would be from the heroin, would it, Doctor?' asked Bulmer.

'That's what we thought at first,' Dr Holmes finally responded. 'But we've just had the results back. Simon Reed also has TB but much much worse than Mr Cassidy. He has fungating TB combined with severe lung disease from excessive use of heroin. Add this to his general ill health from his living conditions and poor diet, his unbalanced state of mind – it is safe to say he is not a well man.'

'There's something else,' I said. They all turned and looked at me. 'Mr Cassidy's son was seeing a nurse. I heard people say Alice Murray was seeing a married man.'

The policeman tutted as he wrote this down.

'And Mr Reed, well, he had a thing about blondes.'

'Don't we all,' brayed the policeman, nudging Dr Holmes, who stepped away from him and back to Sister's side.

I continued. 'And I noticed the black dressing gown cord next to Alice when we found her. That's the same as the one we gave to Mr Reed.'

'I think you'll find, young lady, that hundreds of men have black dressing gown cords. That sort of clue is more The Famous Five than Bethnal Green,' said Detective Constable Bulmer, pleased with his little joke at my expense.

'Hadn't you better go and actually look for these men and find out who tried to strangle Alice Murray rather than insult my nursing staff?' scolded Sister.

Dr Holmes grinned. 'I think we've helped you as best we can, Detective Constable. Let me walk you out.'

The night passed uneventfully but it seemed a nervousness had seeped into every patient. It was as if, rather than infecting their inmates with TB, Mr Cassidy and Mr Reed had passed on their restlessness to the entire ward. No one slept well, men were up and down all night needing the loo, wanting pain relief, or more food or water. So by the time the sun came up I couldn't wait for my shift to be over and get to my own bed.

By five o'clock most patients had finally drifted off to sleep. I went to the kitchen to make myself a cup of tea. I didn't care if I got into trouble, I needed it – I'd been on my feet for a solid ten hours. As I came back onto the ward, illicit cup and saucer in hand, I noticed the light shining from Mr Cassidy's room. I crept over and to my amazement there he was with his son and heir, Charlie Cassidy. Charlie was helping his old man into his pyjamas and dressing gown, the pair of them smoking cigars and unsteady on their feet, clearly the worse for drink.

'Mr Cassidy, where have you been?' I barked.

'Nurse, I've been with my boy to see our fighter. Couldn't miss it; we had our shirts riding on him, but it paid off, didn't it, Charlie Boy,' bellowed Old Man Cassidy, slapping Charlie on the back.

'Mr Cassidy, the police are looking for you,' I told him.

'The police? You can't send the police for a man who takes himself off for a few hours – it's not a crime to have a bit of fun, is it?'

'You didn't tell anyone where you were going,' I explained.

'Well, you'd have said no,' he snorted as he helped himself to another Scotch right in front of me.

'Yes, we would, because you're infectious, Mr Cassidy.'

'Infectious?' said Charlie, jumping back. 'What's he got?'

'TB,' I said rather pertly.

'Oi, that's my business,' shouted Mr Cassidy.

'Not when you are putting others at risk,' I informed him. 'And not when you go missing at the same time there's been a very serious assault on a nurse in the hospital grounds.'

'What's that got to do with me?' roared Mr Cassidy.

He and Charlie, who'd been as thick as thieves when I'd come in, were now at opposite ends of the room.

'Did either of your know Alice Murray?' I asked.

'Alice,' said Charlie. 'What's happened to Alice?'

'I think you should ask the police that question,' I responded, not wanting to give away too much – he could be the assailant for all I knew.

'Tell me,' shouted Charlie, coming fast towards me with the same vicious face I'd seen when he'd punched his brother's lights out on Infants Ward.

I jumped out of the way and he thundered into the wall. I quickly opened the door and bolted it, locking father and son in together. I ran to telephone the porters for help. I heard Charlie screaming at his father, 'What have you got your goons to do to my Alice?'

I was so tired when I finally finished my shift but I couldn't face the nurses' dining room, the banter and the theories about what had happened to poor Alice Murray. The porters had called Night Sister and she had called the police. We discovered the Cassidys had been running bare-knuckle fights – the whole gang had been there, and even one or two policemen, so they all had an alibi. Old Man Cassidy couldn't have cared less about his son's adultery as long as he remained faithful to the family business. It was just a horrible, horrible coincidence that Alice had been seeing Charlie Cassidy. He'd gone to her bedside as soon as the police had finished with him. Thankfully, she'd regained consciousness in the early hours but was unable tell us who had done it; she told the police she'd never even seen her attacker. He'd come up on her from behind and wrapped the cord around her neck; all she'd heard was rambling cries about family, and heroin, and coffee and cornflakes.

I took a stroll round the hospital grounds; at eight o'clock in the morning it was still fairly quiet and the rain had only just stopped. I left through the side gate and crossed over the road to St Barnabas. I didn't know if the church would be open but I needed a sanctuary, a quiet place to unravel my thoughts about that hideous night before I could even attempt to sleep. As I heavily trod the wet path to the church doors, there, lying on a tombstone under the baleful eyes of an angel, like an errant homing pigeon, was Simon Reed, still dressed in his sodden pyjamas and green dressing gown. There was no cord to tie it. I knelt down and felt for his pulse; it was so faint he was barely breathing, and he was so cold it was like he was already dead. I banged on the church doors, the Church Warden came to my aid and we carried this lost soul to Casualty. Simon was barely conscious; he couldn't speak through all the coughing and wheezing.

We'd just got him onto the bed in Casualty when his breathing stopped completely. Charge Nurse Andrews swept me aside but he couldn't find a pulse. He began cardiac massage but it was all too late. Simon had a cardiac arrest and died within minutes. I hoped he found peace.

16

I felt sticky and uncomfortable as I walked alone from the bus stop at Finsbury Park towards Alex's maisonette. It had been a dull and rainy August, but September 1971 was an Indian summer. The streets were burning under my tired expanding feet, the air was dry and my head was all fuzzy. The close weather was making everyone irritable. We shuffled along the hot pavement next to overcrowded smelly buses and cars with exasperated drivers tooting their horns, their windows wound down, cigarette smoke billowing out to mix with the humid air. My new cream linen minidress was sticking to the back of my thighs and my feet were aching already in my new strappy sandals. I'd bought this extravagant ensemble, covered in leaves and flower-shaped buttons in a mix of pink, tan and royal blue, to wear for my homecoming.

Alex had borrowed his dad's Hillman Minx to drive us from Hackney to my parents' house in Wales. He'd been embarrassed by the somewhat dated four-door saloon but I knew nothing about cars and didn't understand what he was apologising for – to me a car was the same as any other, something to take you from A to B. As we cruised along the highway on the last weekend of August, singing along to Mungo Jerry's 'In the Summertime', I felt light and happy. The cool sea breeze was a welcome relief for both of us. I smooched up next to Alex on the beige leather seats, his arm around my shoulders; as we twisted and turned down country lanes he told me, 'I'd do anything for you, Sarah.'

But then something had changed; I was now haunted by the shock on his face as we drove up the hill to Uplands and he took in the size of the house and land. I'd never said much about my family or the house because I knew it was never going to be my home again – when I was in Hackney my parents' house was a distant memory, like school or bucket-and-spade holidays – relegated to my childhood past. I was just a student nurse, a girl in love for the first time – I didn't think that money mattered as long as you had enough to eat and a roof over your head.

All too painfully, though, I was now realising it was easy for money not to matter when you had it, but for Alex it mattered – it really mattered. His words stung me when we'd joined my brothers and sisters in the unoccupied flat above the stables to listen to music and drink cider late into the evening. He said almost seriously, 'We could live in the stables – they're twice the size of my dad's flat.' He made a joke of it and we laughed but he was thoughtful and even quieter than usual. Or was I reading too much into it; was he actually testing the waters? He'd talked often enough about us living together in some rural idyll.

We'd had a fun time at the seaside, and family meals were always sumptuous and raucous, but since we'd driven back to London I'd not heard a word from Alex. When I rang the flat, his brothers or his dad always told me he was out. Right now, I was on my way to have it out with him, because if he didn't want to see me any more I thought I at least deserved to be told so to my face. Okay, maybe I should have said a little bit more about my family background, but he didn't exactly spill the beans on his. Why should it matter to him that he didn't have any money? it didn't matter to me. What sort of reason was that to chuck someone who loves you, who really loves you? I was getting crosser and crosser with each step.

Alex's brother Andy let me in as he was leaving. I entered the small, slightly old-fashioned, simply furnished living room to find Alex all alone, sitting on the old brown sofa watching *Top of the Pops* with Carole King singing 'It's Too Late' gently in the background. The rest of the family were out for once, and he wouldn't even turn his head to look at me when I came in.

'Why haven't you rung me, Alex?'

He didn't say anything, just kept his eyes fixed on the TV, while I stood behind the sofa staring at the back of his head. He was so close, I wanted to reach out and touch him, kiss him, shake him, make him see sense. I longed for him to look me, touch me, press me close to him, but there was just silence and a big empty space between us. Defeated by his refusal to engage, I felt all the anger draining away and in its place was a desperate sadness. Why won't he look at me, why won't he speak to me? 'Is it over, Alex?' I asked. I only saw the back of his head nod and the silence went on and on. In the end I slipped away and walked desolated back to the nurses' home, tears stinging my eyes in the heat of the early evening. He didn't ring, he didn't write – I never saw him again.

The stifling heat went on and on and I struggled to sleep at night in the muggy atmosphere of the nurses' home. I lay awake in my small bed, thoughts of Alex turning over and over in my mind, and hugged myself until fitful sleep eventually came in the early hours of the morning. I decided I would throw myself into my work on the Gynaecological Ward – it was a relief to be consumed with other people's problems and to not have the time or the energy to think about my own. And if ever there was a ward that put you off the idea of marriage and babies it was this one. It felt like women's lives were reduced to their reproductive function as we comforted woman after woman enduring the loss of children that would never be, following hysterectomies, or children that could not be, after abortions.

Gynae was a thirty-five bed ward with two neat rows of patients from top to bottom. Stretching out into the distance were a mix of women from teenagers to octogenarians, of all classes, colours and circumstances, married and unmarried. It made my break-up with Alex seem tiny compared to the physical and emotional trauma so many of these women were enduring. I was glad to have both Maddox and Daniels working on the ward with me, but there was also Prendergast again. She'd been put on 1 to 10 pm shifts with me for the first week while Maddox and Daniels had the best shift of all, 8 am to 4 pm, which was like having an afternoon off. It was sickening to watch Prendergast fawn over the two consultants during morning rounds, not that either Mr Ridley or Mr Mellor would have given a second look to a girl like her.

Both doctors would do only what was absolutely essential, then say, 'I'm on call,' and disappear off to Harley Street for the rest of the day, leaving the work to each of their registrars and housemen. The consultants' bitter rivalry in both NHS and private practice caused a great deal of trouble when they needed a second opinion – they'd refer to surgeons at the London or Bart's rather than to each other, making the whole process drawn out and not in the best interests of their patients. Rumour was they'd both been crossed in love at Oxford when they'd set their caps at the same girl and both lost. Now, middle aged, balding and growing plump on rich dinners and well-stocked wine cellars, their rancour didn't seem to have lessened with age. I could barely tell one from the other – it must have been like despising your own reflection in the mirror, they were so similar.

Sister had asked me to sit with Mrs Seymour and wait for the registrar to come after an unsatisfactory consultation with Mr Mellor. Hackney born and bred, and just into her seventies, the candid Mrs Seymour saw no reason not to tell Mr Mellor what she thought of his bedside manner. He'd unceremoniously diagnosed her with cancer of the womb after a very terse exchange in which he'd asked her if she experienced any pain during intercourse and she'd replied, 'My Bert's been dead twenty-five years – what you implying?' After that, she'd deliberately passed wind during his attempts at a pelvic exam. Mr Mellor stormed off, his nose wrinkled in disgust, chuntering about the lower orders and informing Sister to bleep Dr Chakravarti to finish the exam.

As we waited for the registrar to take over where Mr Mellor had left off, Mrs Seymour told me, 'I thought I was done with the curse and then the bleeding started again and I knew I wasn't right. When your time's up, it's up. I don't want that doctor and his knife anywhere near my downstairs, you hear me, Nurse.'

I was searching for the words to reassure Mrs Seymour but there were none, and then I saw Dr Chakravarti float in, her white doctor's coat over a bright yellow sari, her long dark hair wound up in a coiled bun. She was tall and elegant and moved with grace across the ward. She didn't wait for Sister but came directly to Mrs Seymour's bedside and said, 'Good afternoon, Mrs Seymour. I'm sorry to keep you waiting.'

The old lady didn't say anything. She was shocked – an Indian doctor and a woman at that. She managed a tight-lipped, 'Hullo.'

'Nurse, I'm absolutely parched. Would you mind getting me and Mrs Seymour a cup of tea?' politely requested Dr Chakravarti.

I was taken aback. I hurried off to fetch them a brew and when I returned Dr Chakravarti was sitting next to Mrs Seymour, not standing over her talking at her but listening to her and laughing gently.

'Ah, thank you, Nurse,' she said smoothly as she took her cup. 'Mrs Seymour and I have just discovered we both share a passion for Clark Gable films,' she explained as she sipped her tea. 'Hmm, that's just what the doctor ordered,' she said appreciatively. 'Now, Mrs Seymour, after we've finished our tea I'm going to do a pelvic exam. It won't hurt but it may be a bit uncomfortable and I'm going to have to ask some quite personal questions to try and figure out how best we can help you. Is that all right?'

'You do what you need to, love, and ask away – I've got nothing to hide,' answered Mrs Seymour as she bit down on a bourbon biscuit.

After they finished Dr Chakravarti took me to one side and asked me to keep her informed of how Mrs Seymour was doing. 'A positive state of mind is the most important thing of all. I think the cancer has spread and there is very little we can do for her but minimise her pain and keep her spirits up. What do you think, Nurse Hill?'

Again, I was taken aback – a doctor talking to me, let alone asking my opinion, was unheard of. 'I think you're right, Doctor. Doing little things to ensure patients feel like the people they are and not just their condition is so important,' I replied.

'I have some film magazines at home; perhaps if Mrs Seymour can no longer go to the pictures we can bring a little bit of movie magic to her?' suggested Dr Chakravarti.

'I could read them to her. I think her eyesight isn't very good,' I agreed.

'Splendid,' said the doctor as she floated off to check on another patient.

Sister came and joined me; I think I may have been standing there slightly opened mouthed. 'She'll go far,' said Sister. 'Nurse Hill, I want you to ensure you pay particular attention tonight to Miss Fields; she's just had a very long termination by drip and is in a bad way.'

'An abortion, Sister?'

'Yes, Nurse, an abortion. Daniels assisted but she finishes at four o'clock and I want you to take over when they bring Miss Fields through to the ward – do you have a problem with that?'

'No, Sister,' I answered, but in truth I didn't know the answer – I'd never had to think about something like that. Poor girl, poor baby.

'Good. We are not here to judge, Nurse Hill. We are here to care. Remember Florence Nightingale said, "Every patient in this house is an honoured guest." Daniels will let you know the situation so far; she's disposing of the foetus.'

The New Arrival

Sister was right. Florence Nightingale was right. I felt cross with myself that I'd been so shocked. I went off to find Daniels to try and find out a bit more about the situation. I discovered her on her own in the sluice room with the foetus laid out on a white sheet. Daniels was holding a bowl of water and sprinkling droplets onto its head. I watched her silently as she blessed it by making a sign of the cross on its forehead with her thumb.

'What are you doing?' I asked her.

'I couldn't let the child go without baptising it first. Who knows, one day he might meet his mother in heaven,' she told me. Her face was wet with tears.

I looked down at the tiny still body before me. 'Does she know it was a boy?' I asked.

Daniels shook her head. 'No, she never saw it. She didn't say a word the whole time, not one word, and now it's all over she's got to pick herself up and carry on as if he never was. And she's got no one; she's not much more than a child herself.'

As soon as dinner was over the majority of the nursing staff went, leaving me with Prendergast for the night. But once ten o'clock came my fellow student nurse was nowhere to be seen. I had to attend to every bed on my own, and with thirty-five beds that was a lot of running up and down. Just where was she? I complained to myself as I ran from bed to bed – trust Prendergast to shirk her duties. A little after midnight things started to settle down and there were just two women still awake, Mrs Pinner and Miss Fields. Mrs Pinner was reading by a small torch so she wouldn't disturb her neighbours. She'd come in for a hysterectomy but seemed to be recovering well.

'Can I get you anything, Mrs Pinner?' I whispered.

'No, dear, I'm happy reading. I don't get the time for it much; my four boys keep me pretty busy. It's practically a luxury to be in the company of women and get to read uninterrupted something that I'm not teaching for A-level English,' she said with a low laugh.

'What are you reading?' I asked. Oh, come on now, Sarah. You're delaying going to check on Miss Fields, you coward, I scolded myself.

'*The Hobbit*,' said Mrs Pinner. 'I'm nearly done; I'll leave it for you to read. It's very, very good.'

'Thank you,' I said as I crept away. I made my way over to Miss Fields's bed. She was curled up on one side looking at the wall, wide awake but unnaturally still.

'Can I get you anything?' I now finally asked her in a stifled whisper. She didn't say anything; she rolled over and looked at me with huge glassy blue eyes. Her dark brown curls were tied up with a powder-blue ribbon into a pony tail. She wore a loose-fitting long blue-and-white check nightdress. She looked like a little doll, so tiny in the bed and lost in the vast ward.

I scurried off to the kitchen and put some toast on and made two cups of tea and popped to the linen cupboard to get some fresh knickers and sanitary pads. I returned with the tea and toast on a tray and sat down beside her. I smiled and said, 'I'm starving, aren't you? We're not supposed to eat on the wards, but who doesn't break the rules these days?' She sat up slowly and reached out for the cup of tea. 'There's some strawberry jam in the cupboard – fancy some of that on your toast?' She nodded. When I came back she'd eaten all her portion so I put the jam on mine and gave her the plate.

'What about you?' she asked in a small voice.

'I'll get some in a bit. You eat up.' I sat next to her until she'd finished. 'Would you like me to take you to the loo?' I asked.

She nodded. Once we came back I just sat next to her, holding her small hand until she fell asleep at about four o'clock in the morning. I was just leaving her side to check on the other patients when I saw Prendergast sneak back onto the ward.

'Where have you been?' I asked her.

'I don't have to explain myself to you, Hill.'

'I've had thirty-five patients to attend to on my own all night.'

'If you're not up to the job, it's not my fault.'

'You're lucky nothing serious happened,' I warned her.

'Looks like you had nothing better to do than sit with that strumpet,' she said slyly, waving a dismissive hand at Miss Fields's bed.

'You shouldn't talk about patients like that, Sister says …'

'Teacher's pet now, are we? I didn't become a nurse to look after the likes of her. Most of the women on this ward are no better than they ought to be, that's why they are here.'

'What utter rubbish,' I hissed.

'Why so sensitive? Boyfriend chucked you and left you in the family way too?' She sneered and then flounced off to the kitchen. Oh, I was mad, but I was even madder the next night when she did it again, and the next. Just what was she up to?

Me, Maddox and Wade were in our usual corner of the Adam & Eve. I'd finally finished my week of night duty and was going onto the 8 am to 4 pm shift. Prendergast had left me in the lurch all week and on the last night I'd had enough.

'So, what did you say to her when she eventually turned up?' asked Maddox.

'I'd told her Matron had done a surprise inspection and asked where she was, and I'd been forced to tell Matron that Prendergast had been abandoning her post all week.'

'No. What did she do?' gasped Wade.

'She went as white as a sheet and for the first time ever she was speechless. I told her she was to report immediately to Night Sister to explain herself. She looked like she'd been told she was for the gallows. I watched her do the dead man's walk all the way to Night Sister's office. Then I called her back just before she was about to knock on the door and told her I'd covered for her this time but I wouldn't do it again.'

'Ha, and did Matron do a surprise inspection?' asked Wade.

'No, I made it up,' I replied.

'You should report her,' Maddox told me.

'Hill's not a grass,' hissed Wade.

Maddox shook her head. I hastily sipped my vodka and lime. Maddox was right: I should have reported her, but snitching just wasn't my thing, though I didn't believe for one minute my little trick would put a stop to Prendergast's ways.

'Have you checked with Alf if it's still all right to hold the meeting upstairs tonight?' asked Maddox. 'I want to put a poster up on the front door.'

'I think he's fine, but I'll check,' I reassured her as I made my way over to the bar. Maddox was nervous – she was holding her own official branch meeting for the Women's Liberation Movement. Who knew if anyone would come?

'Alf, are we still on to have the meeting upstairs tonight?' I asked the burly landlord as he was pulling a pint.

'I never could say no to a nurse,' he replied, giving me a wink.

'We're going to set up; would you direct people upstairs?' I asked and then added under my breath, 'If anyone comes.'

I reported back to Maddox. 'Alf says it's fine.'

'Good. Here, put these posters up and give out these leaflets. I'm going to set the room up,' instructed Maddox as she thrust all her pamphlets at me and bustled off upstairs.

'Give me a read,' said Wade, snatching a leaflet off me as soon as Maddox was out of sight. She hastily read it, her mouth dropping open as she did. 'Well I never; have you read this? It's filthy – I wouldn't have thought Maddox would have it in her.'

'No,' I replied. 'I haven't had a chance yet.'

'Should be an interesting meeting,' said Wade, raising a highly arched brow. 'I think if she'd put on the posters in the nurses' home that we'd be discussing "Women and sex as explored in *The Female Eunuch*" there would have been standing room only by now.'

I shook my head in amusement and put up the posters. Wade made a sudden conversion to Women's Lib and started giving out leaflets and discussing the topic of the evening at the bar – though I wasn't sure she understood who our audience was as I saw her write down a few phone numbers from a group of porters and one or two doctors. I decided not to mention it to Maddox and removed myself from the situation by running upstairs to see if the room was ready.

The upstairs room was cosier than the saloon bar. It had the same tree-patterned wallpaper peeling at the edges and stained yellow from tobacco, and the same thick smell of beer, smoke and sweat tinged with disinfectant and wood polish, but here the world outside wasn't as easily forgotten as it was in the shadowy bar below. A big oval window lit the room from the back so you stood eye to eye with the passengers on the red double-decker buses as they passed by.

Maddox had predictably arranged the chairs in neat utilitarian rows facing a central table at the front, where she was now setting up her papers and stacks of copies of the book in question.

'Maddox, it's very well organised … only it's not a hustings; it's a discussion group. We want women to share their stories, ideas and concerns. I don't think organising us like we're in one of Sister Connors's lectures is going to get the conversation flowing,' I told her.

Maddox scowled, 'What would you suggest instead?'

'Let's move the tables out of the way and put the chairs in a circle.'

Maddox thought for a moment. 'All right, take the other end of this table,' she told me as we started hauling more furniture about. The meeting was due to start in ten minutes and it was still just me, her and now Wade representing the women's cause for Hackney General's nurses' home.

The inner circle of our first meeting consisted of me, Maddox, Wade, Patel and some midwives Wade knew from the Mothers' Hospital – a Mauritian girl called Luck and a Scottish girl called Macleod. Like me, the other girls had a drink and a few curled-up sandwiches kindly laid on by Alf's wife Maureen. I tried to convince the landlady to join us but she'd told me, 'All a bit late for me now, lovey. If I start thinking too much about my lot I'd probably leave him, and then where would I be? Don't fancy kipping under the arches at my age.'

We each skim-read the materials Maddox had brought until we felt sufficiently relaxed to sit down and have a discussion. We looked at the floor and then from face to face, not quite knowing what to do.

'We need to consider what our demands are,' announced Maddox.

'I demand another drink,' tittered Wade.

The other girls laughed. Maddox ignored her and continued. 'If we look at the discussion on work in the book, you can see the inequality between men and women in the workplace is laid out with all the figures,' began Maddox in a high, nervous voice. We all tutted in agreement, having been involved in an unfair pay dispute ourselves, and Maddox's voice returned to its normal pitch as she found her theme. 'Also the assumption that women only work until they have children is just not true. The Man wants to split married and unmarried women so they can rule us.'

'You don't have to be married to be a mother,' Luck teased Maddox.

'No, of course not,' agreed Maddox, reddening. 'But women need greater choice on if they become mothers and wives at all – it should not be a *fait accompli*.'

'Are you talking about Free Love?' asked Patel with a tinge of disgust in her voice.

'In my experience love's never free,' jibed Wade.

'I'm talking about free choice,' Maddox explained.

'But it's only cleaners and factory workers and seamstresses that keep working once they're married or *unmar-*

ried with kids,' said Macleod. 'You don't see professional women like nurses carrying on once they're married. Matron, all the Sisters, Staffs, they haven't a husband between them and I don't want to end up like them.'

'Like Matron, oh no,' giggled Patel. 'Get to me to the church now.'

Maddox glared at Patel and Macleod as they twittered.

'It shouldn't be one thing or the other,' I said. 'Why can't women have a job that fulfils them and have a family if they want to?'

'Exactly,' said Maddox enthusiastically. 'I believe there are two things that we should demand. One is access to free childcare and the other is free access to contraception.'

This room of predominantly unmarried, childless girls looked perplexed. There was silence and we all started to fidget, looking either guilty or very uncomfortable at the turn of the conversation.

'As the only woman who has been married and had a child, can I tell you something,' interjected Wade. 'You girls would benefit much more from the chapters that tell you about sex and getting the pill before you start worrying about marriage and babies.'

'Edie!' I gasped.

'Now, access to free contraception, that's worth having,' said Wade. 'Any of you unmarried girls tried to get the pill?'

I shook my head instantly and looked at Maddox, who had a scarlet rash spreading from under her collar right up to her forehead.

'I went to Woollies and bought myself a wedding ring,' whispered Macleod.

'I told them I was getting married in a month,' giggled Luck.

'Why should you have to lie? The biggest lie in the world is that unmarried women don't have sex,' shouted Wade.

'Yes, but isn't going on the pill just giving men a free ride to get what they want?' said Patel primly.

'And what about what you want?' Wade asked, arching her brow.

Patel looked at her highly polished black court shoes.

'Yes, but no one will want to marry you if they think you've slept around,' Macleod stated.

'Marriage is just a prison for women,' Maddox said to no one.

'Gynae ward is full of women with unwanted pregnancies, both married and unmarried,' I said. 'It's more than just taking a pill – it's women's state of mind that needs to be opened up. It's not just unmarried women who have unwanted babies.'

'You're telling that to a midwife, Hill. Do you know how many mothers of five, six, seven or more have asked me to tie their tubes after delivery? Offered to slip a fiver into my pocket if I'll make sure they'll never have another baby. I could've had a fur coat by now. And I'm tempted, not for the money, but because they're slaves to their reproduction. Slaves to this part of the body that can't be mentioned in polite company, that most men barely understand despite the amount of time they spend there,' Wade finished breathlessly.

'So are we agreed?' asked Maddox. 'We demand along with our Sisters in the Women's Liberation Movement that all women should have free access to contraception. Say Aye.'

We all cried 'Aye' and raised our hands.

'Maddox, there's something in this talking business,' Wade enthused. 'I thought it would just be a load of ugly girls banging on about how they can't win a beauty competition.'

It was with feelings of ferocious feminism that I walked into the hospital the next morning and saw little Miss Fields sitting alone in the lobby waiting to be picked up. The poor girl should have been discharged days ago but she'd had some bad bleeding and been kept in. She was hunched on one side of the bench, her hand on her empty tummy circling round and round where her baby should have been, staring at the double doors – waiting.

'Hello,' I said softly. 'Going home this morning?' She nodded. 'Is someone picking you up?' She nodded again. I looked at the clock: it was only 7.50 am – surely they'd not discharged her so early?

'I don't think he's coming,' she whispered.

'It's not even eight o'clock yet. Have you had breakfast?' She shook her head. 'What's the rush to get off so early?'

'They let me go last night,' she told me as her hand reached up to her chest to suppress a sob.

'You've been sitting here all night?' I was so shocked.

'He said he'd pick me up,' she said once more.

'The father?' I asked.

'Not now he ain't. He dropped me off here quick enough. He said he'd come back for me – he promised.'

'Have you rung him?' I asked.

'He won't let me,' I looked at her blankly. 'In case his wife answers,' she explained.

'Oh. Where do you need to get to?'

'Home, the King Henry's Walk. My ma thinks I'm staying at my friends. I'll have to wander about till school's out and then get the bus, I suppose.'

Poor girl, and now I had to face what I'd known all along: Miss Fields was only a schoolgirl, an innocent child, and she'd had to cope with all this on her own; all the dirty looks from the auxiliaries, the whispers behind her back from the other patients, the dismissive doctors. What choice did she have in all of this? I knew then that the decision forced onto her – whether to be a mother or not – came too late. Girls needed to know they had a choice about whether to have sex or not and, if they did, how to keep themselves safe. Maddox was right, women and girls needed free access to contraception and they needed educating, and I needed to educate myself too. I knew nothing, nothing at all.

I looked into my purse. All I had was two pounds and a sixpence. I quickly took out the two pounds and pressed it into her hand so no one would see.

'If you need somewhere to stay till school's out, go across the road to St Barnabas and ask for Gerald. Just say Sarah Hill sent you, and you need a breakfast and lunch and somewhere to rest. Then use this two pounds for a taxi home; you're in no fit state to get the bus,' I told her. Miss Fields stared amazed at the money in her hand. I smiled at her and patted her knee. 'Go,' I instructed, tilting my head in the direction of the door.

I watched her steadily walk out of the hospital and into the church, then I went and did my shift. I didn't tell anyone, it didn't matter whether they praised or censured me – I didn't want to hear it. I was just beginning to understand that a woman needs two things if she's going to stand a chance of a happy life: her health and an education, and we had a long way to go on both those fronts as far as I could see.

17

I stood surveying the half-emptied boxes with my cup of tea in hand. The morning light was just starting to make its way through the thin curtains into the threadbare room. Bottles and plates lay abandoned on the upturned cardboard boxes we'd used as tables to consume our first meal in our new home.

Maddox had found the flat on the Balls Pond Road only two weeks before, after seeing it advertised on a card in the newsagent's window. We and Lynch had moved in with a lot of haste and excitement, pooling our meagre wages to pay for a cramped, unmodernised top-floor flat. For our first meal I'd cooked lamb chops and veg in some tiny saucepans I'd bought at Woollies and I served it up on an assortment of crockery I was given by Pearl from Infants Ward. She'd kindly passed on a black oval serving dish and four plastic melamine plates, bowls and cups and saucers. Three unwashed mugs still held the remnants of the cheap wine Lynch had bought, and we'd toasted ourselves long into the night.

I'd had a restless night on the nylon sheets that our land-lord had provided, and as I made up my single bed with

'What?' I was perplexed.

'I'll explain later. Tea in the laundry around one o'clock while the visitors are in?'

'Looking forward to it already,' I smiled.

It was so good to be working with Appleton again. Of course we'd met up; gone to the pictures and London Zoo, we'd even seen Margot Fonteyn in the ballet and Ingrid Bergman in the West End, but days off were so few and far between. I'd get to see her all the time now, and it was just what I needed after Alex, after Gynaecology and all the upset of the last few months. I felt that with the babies and toddlers was where I belonged.

My first glimpse of Paul Murphy, the boy with Perthes disease, filled me with pity for the poor little lad. The loss of bone mass had damaged his femur, resulting in a very bad limp, and his leg was in traction to give the blood vessels at the hip and socket a chance to heal. It was a long-drawn-out treatment that had already lasted for months. You couldn't help but feel for him lying there day after day unable to leave the bed. He was sharing his room with a mischievous freckle-faced three-year-old called Richie Turnball. This little scamp was the youngest of six brothers, always getting into scrapes. I'd met at least two of his older siblings previously when they'd been brought in for broken limbs. Now little Richie had joined the club after falling onto to the tarmac and bumping his head as a result of shinning down the drainpipe from an upstairs window.

Right now he was completely occupied building a tower of biscuits.

'Hello, I'm Nurse Hill. How are you feeling today, Paul?' I asked as I took his notes down from the wall.

'I'm bored,' he said meekly. 'I miss my mum,' he sniffed.

'Will she be in to see you later?'

'She comes every day,' he told me, brightening up just a little.

'Oh good,' I said with a sigh of relief. 'Well, we'll just have to find a game to play until she comes. What do you like to play?'

'Snap,' he told me, producing a deck of cards from underneath his pillow.

'That's my favourite card game too,' I told him. 'Do you want to deal the cards for me while I do your pulse and temperature and then we'll have a game?' He nodded enthusiastically. 'Now, let's pop this thermometer under your arm while I take your pulse. How's your leg feeling?'

'Itchy.'

'I'll get you some cream to settle it down, and give you a wash with some water and a flannel. That'll help you feel better. Anything else?'

'I get sharp pains sometimes but most of the time it's very achy. I feel tired even though I ain't doing nothing. My bones aren't right,' he told me with such earnestness for a small boy. I looked at his chart; he was the oldest child on the ward but he was only just five.

I jotted Paul's temperature, pulse and respiration down, made my notes and took the thermometer from under his arm, as he continued dealing out the cards. We played all morning, only pausing briefly for doctors' rounds and lunch. Sometimes Richie joined in but he would only play for a few minutes and then find another game. Before we knew it was almost one o'clock.

'Knock, knock,' said a cheerful voice.

I saw a woman in a green polo neck and tartan miniskirt in the doorway. Her hair was the same shade of sandy brown as Paul's.

'Mummy!' shouted Paul with excitement.

'And how's my baby?' she asked as she raced over to his bed and gave him a hug.

'Mrs Murphy?' I enquired.

'Yes, dear. Nurse …?'

'Hill. Pleased to meet you. Paul's been beating me at snap all morning.'

'That's my boy,' said Mrs Murphy as she wiped a smear of lipstick from her son's cheek. 'I know I'm a bit early,' she said to me in a conciliatory whisper. 'But I missed my Paul so much, I couldn't wait any longer.'

'Don't worry about it. What harm does an extra few minutes do? None. I think it does the children good to have more time with their parents.'

'Don't you let Sister Nivern hear you talk like that, Nurse,' warned Mrs Murphy playfully.

'Oh, no. Quite,' I agreed.

I remembered Sister's words of warning about visiting times and mothers – I was pretty sure Sister Skinflint and Mrs Murphy had already had a run-in. I'm not sure I would have dared contradict her before, but now I knew that other Sisters had a more relaxed attitude to visitors and the benefit seeing loved ones had on patients. I didn't want to get into trouble, but I wasn't afraid of Sister Nivern any more. Once you've had a run-in or two with Matron and lived to tell the tale, Sister Skinflint didn't look half so scary.

Mrs Murphy stroked Paul's head thoughtfully. 'I come every day. I'd stay with him all the time if I could,' said the doting mama.

'I miss you, Mummy,' said Paul in a small voice.

'I know you do. I miss you too baby, so, so much,' Mrs Murphy soothed her son.

I didn't want to get in the way, and once Mrs Turnball arrived with her brood I took the opportunity to nip out and meet Appleton for our illicit brew in the laundry. Once we were nicely settled down I asked her what was she on about – the mystery of Sister Skinflint's egg sandwich.

'Oh, that,' chuckled Appleton. 'Sister's taken to escaping for half an hour away from prying eyes in the linen cupboard. Every day Pearl has to leave her a cup of tea and an egg sandwich cut into delicate triangles with the crusts cut off. Only, for the last few days when Sister's arrived to indulge herself the sandwich is gone. She's just found crumbs on the linen. Old Skinflint's ever so cross, but of course it's a secret that she's doing it so she can't make a fuss or do a stake-out to find who the culprit is.'

Serves her right, Sister Nivern was always disappearing on little breaks or urgent meetings.

At the end of visiting hours I returned to find Mrs Murphy was still there tearing out a picture from the newspaper she'd been reading to Paul.

'Nurse, would you mind if I put this up for my Paul?' She held up a cutting of the Fab Four. 'My Paul loves the Beatles, they're his favourite band.'

'I don't see why not,' I said.

Paul's face lit up. 'My mum bought me "Octopus's Garden" and "Yellow Submarine" to cheer me up when I came into hospital,' he told me.

'That's kind of her,' I said as he eagerly produced the records from under his pillow to show me.

'Only you don't have a record player, so I haven't heard them,' he said sadly as his fingers held tightly onto his precious records.

'I did try and sneak my record player in,' confessed Mrs Murphy. 'Only Sister Nivern saw me and sent me packing.'

'Do you like the Beatles?' Paul asked me.

I nodded.

'Who's your favourite?' he asked, leaning forward, his leg swinging in the air.

'George. Who's yours?'

'Paul, of course,' he said in surprise at my lack of astuteness.

'Of course,' I said, tutting at myself as Mrs Murphy laughed softly.

'It's so hard for him. He's missed so much,' said Mrs Murphy in a quiet voice as Paul got out a little scrapbook with newspaper cuttings of his favourite bands and looked through the well-thumbed pages. 'He stopped being able to jump and kick a ball like the other boys, but we could still dance around the living room together and enjoy the music. Just the two of us. He could forget himself for just a little bit, forget the limp, forget the pain sometimes, and just be a happy boy. That's why music means so much to him, but Sister won't let me bring a radio in and it's so dull for him in here.'

'How long has he been in hospital for?'

'Two months,' sighed Mrs Murphy. 'I think we'll be here for another two at least. He has to watch all the other children come and go, and he's still here. Stuck in that bed. It's not fair. It's cruel. I don't know why they can't get me a wheelchair and let me take him out sometimes or even home for a night. How would they like it, stuck in that bed day after day without his toys, without the telly or a bit of music? Without his mummy?' She finished, her last words catching in her throat in a suppressed sob.

'It must be very hard on you both,' I sympathised.

'Still, now we're here, we've got to see it through,' she said with a shrug. 'As long as they fix his leg, we can get over months in bed. What we can't cope with is all the other children calling him Long John Silver for the rest of his life. He was perfect when he was born, but then last year he got a limp. It was just a little limp at first but it got worse and worse. I took him to the doctor. He tells me our Paul's just copying his big brother, playing at pirates, it'll pass, he tells me, thinks I'm just a fussy mother. Then our Paul started to get really bad pains all up his leg. I go back to the doctor. This time he tells me it's growing pains. I knew it wasn't growing pains, I said so, but they never listen. You're just a mother, what do you know? I knew the doctor wasn't right, though, so I brought him here and they did lots of X-rays and he saw lots of different doctors and all the time his limp was getting worse. Then the surgeon, he takes a look. Perthes disease, he says. So, now we're getting somewhere, but it doesn't make it any easier on him. He's just a baby. He just wants to be at home with his mum, and his brother and his record player. And who can blame him?'

'We'll have to see if we can do something to cheer him up,' I said.

'You do that, Nurse. Just make sure Sister doesn't catch you,' smiled Mrs Murphy.

It was already seven o'clock in the evening by the time the bus dropped me off. A crowd disembarked at my stop and I was bumped and tossed about in the frosty night air as people pushed to get through. Once I was out of the crush I walked along the dark street confidently, but I could sense a man too close behind me, echoing my steps as I made my way along the grimy pavement. Then he picked up pace as we passed the churchyard and bumped into me and snatched my handbag right off my arm. He raced off into the grave-yard without a word.

I was stunned for the first few seconds and then I went to shout for help but this was the Balls Pond Road so what was the point? Before we'd even moved in our fellow nurses had delighted in recounting stories about the criminal under-world that operated from here. That's why the rent was so cheap; it was the only place we could afford that was near the hospital. Here, Ronnie and Reggie Kray were whispered about in revered tones despite being behind bars. We'd been told that when their mother Violet walked down the street you'd have thought it was the Queen Mother passing by, the way peopled bowed and scraped.

I was a little bruised but mainly unharmed, so what could I do but I walk home defeated to our new flat. I knew after the last time my bag was stolen on Homerton High Street that there was no point reporting it to the police; they'd almost laughed in my face when I'd gone with Maddox to the police station. Luckily there hadn't been much in my bag; since coming to Hackney this was the third time my bag had been stolen. I'd learnt to only keep the minimum in it, and nothing of any value.

* * *

It was just Lynch in the flat when I got home. She was jabbing at the grill with a wooden spoon and a tea towel, looking fed up. She looked up and saw me and then threw the spoon down in a huff.

'Maddox can clean this up herself. She only went and put cheese on toast on a plastic plate under the grill. The whole thing's melted – we're lucky she didn't set the flat on fire. And then to cap it all she just leaves the whole sorry mess to go to one of her Save the World meetings.'

'That's one of my melamine plates,' I complained as Lynch threw it all into the sink. 'I just had my handbag nicked on the way home,' I told her.

'Oh, lord. Have we any wine left?' I looked in the cupboard and found half a bottle of red and poured us both a mug full. 'Bottoms up,' said Lynch as we clinked mugs. The door-bell rang. 'That better not be another caller for the previous occupants,' huffed Lynch as she went and pulled up the sash window and stuck her head out.

'What do you want?' she shouted down to the street.

'I'm looking for Miss Valance,' I heard a man's voice call back.

'No longer at this address,' snapped Lynch.

'You'll do,' I heard the man say saucily.

'But you won't,' spat Lynch as she slammed the window back down. 'That's the sixth caller for the previous tenants I've had since I got home,' Lynch told me.

'What do they want?' I asked.

'Take a wild guess?' said Lynch, folding her arms and giving me a stern look.

'Oh, no. Not that?'

'Yes, that,' she growled.

'We'll have to put up a sign or something,' I suggested.

'Saying what? This is no longer a house of ill repute?'

We both started to laugh.

'What a day,' I said, absentmindedly flopping down onto the wonky armchair and promptly being tipped out onto the lino. I just lay back flat and stared up at the cracked ceiling. Lynch came and sat down beside me on the floor.

'When's your next day off?' asked Lynch.

'Tuesday,' I replied.

'Mine too. Fancy going shopping up West? We could catch the bus to High Street Kensington, have a wander in the park, maybe a mooch around Notting Hill?'

I definitely fancied that. I'd always wanted to visit Biba but I'd never had the money. Maybe we could just have a little look – window shopping didn't cost anything. I readily agreed. Thoughts of bargain hunting and being just a girl for a day filled my mind as I went to the sink to attempt removing melted cheese and melamine from the grill so I could make my dinner. A bit of West London living was what I needed after a typical day in Hackney.

18

The following Tuesday morning I pulled on my trusty white boots and stared down at my feet, bare knees and tartan miniskirt. They didn't look like my feet or my legs; I was so used to seeing sensible black flat shoes and stocking legs poking out from the skirt of my nurse's uniform. Being in mufti was suddenly foreign, like that was the person I used to be, not me now. For the last few days I'd been working long shifts from dawn till dusk and had tumbled straight into bed when I got back to the flat.

I heard Lynch's footsteps running up the stairs. 'Post's come,' she told me as she re-entered the flat. She already had her coat on over a matching navy miniskirt and jacket. 'One letter for you, two for me, and a stack of pamphlets and lefty communist magazines for Maddox.' She handed me a small pale blue envelope. I recognised my mother's hand immediately. Suddenly I was eager to know everyone was all right. I'd had very little contact with home since driving off into the sunset in Alex's father's Hillman Minx at the end of August. I edged my finger along the flap of the envelope and pulled out my letter.

24th November 1971

Dear Sal [I'd been named Sarah Elizabeth after my paternal grandmother; my mother communicated her feelings about her mother-in-law by calling me Sally.]

I just remembered it was your birthday yesterday – Many Happy Returns of the Day. I often think of you in London and imagine it is much like my time in the Wrens during the war – full of fun, friends, working hard and having a great time – dancing and seeing all the sights, and luckily for you, you don't have bombs dropping all the time interrupting things.

Thanks for sending us a postcard with your new address. Are you sure getting a flat in that area is safe? I guess you haven't had much time for writing lately and neither have I. Your father had us slaving away in the orchards all autumn. I have made enough Victoria plum jam to spread on all the scones at The Oval I should think. We've been making chutney too so the larder is very well stocked. Now, I've got all the preparations for Christmas to do. The puddings and the cake are already done but there are a lot of parties coming up at your father's work.

Old Dai has taken to bringing the milk later than ever and we are lucky to get it before nightfall at the moment. He has no sense of time and brings it on his tractor which tears up the drive making potholes and causing a terrible racket. Your father is not amused either.

Jane has brought a dog home, his previous owner couldn't cope with his nervous temperament and neither can I. He's 'barking' mad and gets loose all the time scaring the goat and

the cats, and if he gets into the farmers' fields he'll be shot.
Good riddance. His name is Freud and he's a Dalmatian which
says it all really. It's totally out of character for her to do some-
thing so impulsive – I don't think art college is having a good
effect on her.

Your father is coming to London to his head office soon for
the company Christmas do, but I can't spare the time as I'm on
the Mothers' Committee at church. He's enclosed a note about
meeting up.

Don't forget if you want to come home at any time just a
note or a telephone call and your room will be waiting for you.
Do try and come for Christmas. And if the new flat is horrid
you don't have to stay there if you don't want to.

Love Mum

I turned the letter over and saw a small square of card with
Dad's name printed on it pinned to the back of the letter. I
tore if off and saw his writing on the back of his business
card.

Meet me at The Dorchester 17th December at 6 pm.
Check your shoes.
Dad

I dropped down to my knees and excitedly pulled out my
old school trunk from underneath my bed. I'd chucked in an
impractical pair of shoes my mother had given me on my
last visit home in the summer. I hadn't bothered to unpack

the snakeskin peep-toed shoes or the matching purse, unnecessary as they were to my new life. I reached my hand inside the left shoe – nothing. I picked up the right shoe and peered into it and tapped the toe. A ten pound note fluttered into my lap. Only my father would hide money in people's shoes for when they might need it. I smiled broadly; bless my dad – he must have been wondering if I'd ever find it. This shopping trip was going to be much more fun now. I'd get a dress I could wear to meet him at The Dorchester, I thought excitedly, one from the Biba shop on High Street Ken.

'Well, thank you, Daddy,' whistled Lynch as I popped the ten pounds into my purse. 'Hill, would you come on; we'll miss the bus.'

I sprang up, grabbing my navy Reefer jacket from the back of the sofa. My coat seemed like a long-lost item too; I'd been wearing my cape to and from the hospital to get free bus rides but today unless Clifford was on we were going to have to pay the fare. Today I wasn't a nurse; today I was out to have a good time.

We hopped off the No. 9 bus just outside High Street Kensington tube station and I gazed up at the towering Biba store in Barkers Arcade. It was ten o'clock in the morning and it felt like the folks of well-heeled Kensington hadn't woken up yet, unlike Hackney which had been buzzing with life even before the sun came up. We'd travelled into town on the top deck of a crowded bus, pressed up against commuters, watching through the windows the bustle of the market traders for whom eight o'clock in the morning was practically lunchtime, and enjoying the sight of gaggles of children skipping along the pavement on their way to school.

Lynch and I linked arms as we walked through the large entrance of the store. The sound of Paul Jones singing 'Aquarius' filled my ears. Everything seemed black with flashes of gold, just like the Biba logo itself. The wallpaper was black with hundreds of tiny bananas on it.

'I think this is the grooviest place I've ever been,' I said to Lynch.

'Me too. It's more like a nightclub than a shop.'

Behind the counter were young, big-eyed and stick-thin girls, just like the Biba models themselves. They were listlessly folding dresses and tops in a deep mauve colour with swirling paisley design all over it.

'Gosh, nice uniform if you can get away with it,' whispered Lynch, as we walked past the counter and the Biba girls in their miniskirts and go-go boots.

'Imagine Matron's face if we cut our uniform down to that short a miniskirt,' I replied.

'I imagine it would look something like this,' she said, dropping her jaw and clutching her heart.

The doe-eyed fawns behind the counter temporarily stopped their folding and looked up with widening eyes at our lack of decorum.

'Maybe we should keep a low profile,' I whispered to Lynch.

'Not a bit,' Lynch brazened, giving them a cheery 'Hello' as she wandered up to a clothes rail filled with new maxi coats and gasped at the price tag.

'They've gone up a fair bit in price since they switched from mail order to a high street fashion house,' said Lynch as she flicked through the coat-hangers one by one.

I smiled. 'So much for affordable fashion for ordinary girls. This is catwalk stuff,' I agreed.

We wandered around until I found some dresses that were more in my price range. Two caught my eye. One was a black minidress in the same pattern as the banana wallpaper, the other was a long black maxi dress with deep cuffs and sleeves that were covered with little buttons all the way up to the elbow.

'That's lovely,' said Lynch as I held the maxi dress up to me and looked in the mirror. 'How much?'

'Five pounds.'

'Can you afford that?'

'No, but my dad can,' I answered sheepishly.

'How much is the other one?'

I looked at the price tag on the mini dress. 'Ten pounds.'

'What ever happened to the twenty-five shilling dress?'

'They've obviously thrown it out along with the shillings,' I retorted, stroking the soft fabric of the banana print. It was the most far-out dress. It was pure swinging London. I'd never had anything so fab. Although my mother was always impeccably dressed herself, I was often a bit threadbare in the wardrobe department since my sisters and I had outgrown the regular visits to Selfridges for our school uniform and party dresses.

'It is a lot of money. Almost a whole month's wages,' I said, still clutching the mini dress with my eager hands.

'Why not think it over and come back after lunch?' said Lynch. 'It'll still be here this afternoon.'

'All right. Where shall we go next?'

'How about a meander round Kensington Gardens? It's sunny, so we could buy some sandwiches and have a frosty picnic on a park bench.'

'Lovely,' I replied and we linked arms once more and breezed out of the store.

After our sandwiches we drifted around Kensington Gardens, past the palace and the round pond and down to Notting Hill Gate. As we passed through the big black gates we almost tripped over an old man standing on the corner, a burnt-down cigarette clenched between his lips as he leant against the railings holding a sign. 'Antique Superstore, Portobello Road', it read.

'Have you ever been to Portobello Road?' asked Lynch.

'Never. You?' She shook her head.

'Let's go,' she said, dragging me over to the other side of the road with barely a look in either direction at the oncoming traffic. Cars beeped at us to get out of the way. 'Picking up stuff your granny would have thrown out is the latest thing,' she told me.

I was still thinking about that black Biba dress with the banana print as we peered at the curios on the market stalls. It was mainly junk, bric-à-brac, tarnished mirrors in decorative frames and bits of old furniture. Then my eyes fell on an old Dansette record player, and I thought of little Paul Murphy with his Beatles records and nothing to play them on. I wandered up to the stall and tried to play it cool, picking up a few bits and bobs and then flicking through some piles of records before looking over the Dansette. I ran my finger over the creamy grey speaker and control knobs on the front of the set, giving them a quick twiddle and checking for dust before flipping the red lid to reveal the black oval sticker with the manufacturer's label 'J & A Margolin Ltd' still proudly stuck to the inside of the lid. Its grey needle was waiting to play a Decca 45 dark blue record with the band's name and single title on it in white type – 'Brown Sugar', The Rolling Stones. The orange and white striped sleeve was in there too. The Dansette was definitely an old model, but it looked like it was in good working order.

'How much do you want for that old record player?' I asked the woman sitting on a high stool nursing a cuppa.

'Two pounds; it'll last you a lot longer than one of those new-fangled things,' she told me.

'No, you may as well buy a gramophone as that,' said Lynch sarcastically.

'You're right. We had that very model in our sitting room when I was toddler in 1954,' I agreed. 'It's ancient. Let's pop down to Woollies and get a new one.'

'You'll pay a lot more for a new one and they don't make 'em like they used to. Give it a year and you'll be buying another one,' the stallholder insisted.

'Hmm, give it a whirl then,' I told her with little enthusiasm. The record player kicked into life and soon the sounds of The Rolling Stones filled our little corner of Portobello Road. 'It doesn't sound too bad,' I said begrudgingly. 'I'll give you 30 pence.'

'A pound.'

'Throw in five records and I'll give you 50 pence.'

'You can have three records,' she said. 'And nothing before 1967 either. Cheek.'

I picked out The Monkees' 'I'm a Believer' and 'Delilah' for Appleton and I insisted on having the Stones record we'd been listening to.

The woman bagged up my purchases and I huffed and puffed, carrying them up the hill of Kensington Church Street.

'Did you think about having to carry that lot all the way back to Hackney on the bus?'

'No,' I answered. 'But it'll be worth it, and I've still got enough money to get that black maxi dress at Biba.' I put the image of the black mini dress with banana print away. 'It'll be more useful than the other one anyway and far more practical; it is winter after all,' I explained, clutching the record player close to my chest.

'I wouldn't have thought a nice boarding school girl like you would know how to haggle,' Lynch said. I could tell she was just a little bit surprised and impressed.

'My mother may be a lady but she's the biggest bargain hunter and never pays a penny more than she has to. She'll put on an old mac, a headscarf and a pair of ancient boots to go down to the harbour and haggle with the fishermen when the boats come in.' I laughed. 'She may live in the manor, but she knows the price of fish.'

'Good on her,' said Lynch.

'Yes,' I said, feeling proud of my mother and her thrifty ways … when I wasn't on the receiving end.

19

The next day I made sure I arrived at the hospital half an hour early so I could sneak my newly purchased Dansette into our secret tea chest in the laundry room. I went to check on Bobbie Fry and Georgie Edwards and found Mrs Fry quietly sitting alone in the room as the boys restlessly napped under the cover of their steam tents. She turned her head slowly as I entered; she looked so defeated. She wasn't even looking at the boys, just staring down at her green court shoes. Each shoe had a strap across the front with a black button at the outer edge. I remembered those shoes from two years ago; only now the soles looked worn down to nothing and the left shoe had lost its button.

'You came to the house once?' said Mrs Fry listlessly.

'Yes, to bring the boys' medicine,' I replied.

'Medicine. It just prolongs it for them. Lengthens their suffering,' she told me. She didn't meet my eye, just stared blankly at the wall.

I was taken aback. I didn't know what to say. The room was silent except for the hissing of the steam kettles. Then I saw Staff Nurse Lennard gesture to me through the window and I stepped outside the room to see her.

'Bobbie Fry stopped breathing last night,' she told me. 'We had to bring the crash team in. He's stable now but very, very weak.'

'Mrs Fry seems in a very bad way, Staff. I think she believes we are just keeping the boys alive but they are going to die.'

'She's probably right,' shrugged Staff.

'Sister has to talk to the Lady Almoner this time. If she can get them out of that house those boys might stand a chance.'

'And who's going to tell her? Your little plan didn't work last time, did it?' said Staff airily. 'Just monitor them closely, Nurse Hill. And report any alternation in their condition immediately. Nurse Patel will relieve you for your break.'

'If I could just talk to Sister,' I implored.

'Get on with your work. You'll never make a nurse, Nurse,' she tutted as she stomped off down the ward corridor to Sister's office.

I glumly returned to the boys and checked on the water in the steam kettles. Mrs Fry was holding the bronchitis medicine in her hand, intently reading the label. When she saw me she put it in her handbag and snapped it shut. I was sure I'd seen the lid of a small bottle of gin inside her bag.

'I'm going to the lav,' she told me as she swept out of the room.

I sat with the boys and thought about the slum they were forced to call home that I'd visited with Appleton two years ago. It wasn't right. Mrs Fry hadn't been a well woman then, and as for now, she seemed completely physically and mentally drained. I wondered how her sister Mrs Edwards was faring; maybe if I could talk to her between us we could work something out. I pictured Mrs Fry's pale face as she'd gazed at the medicine bottle and jumped to my feet. Something wasn't right, I just knew it. I'd learnt to trust my instincts; I knew the face of desperation when I saw it.

'Appleton,' I called. My friend quickly came from the next bay where she was playing with a clutch of infants. 'Watch the boys. I'll explain later.'

I rushed to the visitors' toilets on the ground floor but they were empty. Feeling a little foolish I trudged back up the stairs and went to the nurses' cloakroom just outside the ward. They were empty except for one closed door. I washed my hands and splashed some cool water on my face. As I looked at my reflection in the mirror I could see two green shoes poking out from under the door, one with a button missing.

'Mrs Fry,' I cried, half afraid of the sound of my own voice.

There was no answer. I tried to open the toilet door but it was locked. I dashed to my handbag and took out a penny and put it in the groove of the screw of the locked door. It turned and the door sprung open, revealing Mrs Fry lying semi-conscious on the floor, a scattered bottle of pills and a half-consumed bottle of gin beside her. I ran to the porters and we brought a trolley and rushed her into Casualty. As I handed her over to Charge Nurse Andrews I heard her cry, 'My baby, my baby.'

Filled with fear she'd done something to the boys, I sprinted back to Infants Ward. The boys were awake. Appleton was reading Bobbie a story while he drank water from a beaker. Georgie was having a quick cuddle with his mother, Mrs Edwards; neither child looked like they were in any immediate danger. I quickly told Mrs Edwards what had happened to her sister. She looked horrified but unsurprised that Mrs Fry should try to take her own life.

'What about the baby?' she asked.

'Bobbie looks fine to me, but I'll call doctor to check them over right away,' I replied.

Mrs Edwards shook her head and said with such sorrow, 'She's pregnant, Nurse.'

I was relieved when Patel arrived so I could take my lunch break. I needed it so badly after the morning's drama. It had been a struggle to comfort Mrs Edwards and take care of Georgie and Bobbie. They'd become increasingly aware of the level of distress in the room and we couldn't risk their breathing getting out of control. I had to stay calm for everyone's sake even though inside I was reeling. Charge Nurse Andrews rang from Casualty to let us know that Mrs Fry was stable and being transferred to Female Medical Ward under the care of Dr Holmes.

'Don't worry,' said Appleton as we each sunk down onto a crate in the laundry room. 'Sherlock will take care of her. She'll be fine.'

'We have to go to the Lady Almoner. Damn Sister Nivern, what's the point of being a nurse if you don't save lives when you can?'

'I know,' said Appleton. 'But not today. You need to be calm, get your case together, or she'll just think you're raving.'

'You're right. They are all out of danger for the moment, so let's be thankful for that.'

'Amen,' said Appleton, and we chinked our teacups together and took a long sip of refreshingly hot tea. 'It's not good for the children, all this drama. We need to do something to lift everyone's spirits,' she suggested.

'You're so right,' I agreed as I opened up the crate I'd been neatly perched on. Sister Skinflint was in a lunchtime staff meeting that was going to last for hours, and quite frankly I didn't care if I got into trouble any more. I lifted my recently purchased Dansette out of the crate and turned to Appleton. 'Time to get the party started.'

Mrs Murphy wrapped her multi-coloured chiffon scarf from Woollies around Paul's eyes and gently eased his beloved records out from under his pillow. I tiptoed in clutching my Dansette to my chest, followed like the Pied Piper by small children and babes in nurses' arms. All the little patients and staff from Infants Ward came to enjoy the surprise. I eased up the lid of the record player, slipped 'Octopus's Garden' out of its cover and placed the black record with a picture of a huge green apple on it onto the turntable. I let the needle touch down on the groove and suddenly the whole ward was filled with music. Paul sat straight up in bed, his arms reaching out to the waves of sound.

'Is it, is it my record, Mummy?' he cried out in hope and delight.

But before Mrs Murphy could answer the voice of Ringo Star did it for her and 'I'd like to be, under the sea,' rang out through Infants Ward. Paul pulled the blindfold from his eyes and saw my little red and white Dansette playing his precious record, and all the children and staff cheered. The only smile in the room bigger than Paul's was Mrs Murphy's, who had tears in her eyes. Appleton was dancing round and round in a circle with all the toddlers; even Staff Nurse was swaying with one of the housemen. I hugged myself as I watched Mrs Murphy holding her young son's hands as she danced with him at the side of his bed.

I looked through to Georgie and Bobbie's room and even Mrs Edwards and Patel had taken the boys out of their steam tents momentarily to let them enjoy the music. I thought, what a difference just a small action could make in a patient's life. Yes, there were rules, but sometimes you have to follow your heart. I'm not letting Bobbie and Georgie go back to that house, I'm just not, I vowed to myself. I looked round at all the children dancing – everyone was there, everyone except little Richie Turnball.

Alarmed at his sudden disappearance, I slipped out and went to each bay and looked under every bed and in every cupboard. Then I started to search the sluice, the linen cupboard, the laundry room and the milk kitchen. Panic started to rise in me; where was that child? I was going to have to tell Staff Nurse he was missing and stop the party, call his mother and conduct a full search for him, and then I noticed the tiniest trail of crumbs going from the linen cupboard to the laundry room. I'd already checked the crates Appleton and I used for our stash of biscuits but I hadn't looked behind the huge laundry baskets. And sure enough, as I tiptoed round to the little space between the basket and the wall, I discovered a little den made with freshly washed blankets and a freckle-faced Richie. He was devouring an egg sandwich with a huge smile and plenty of egg all over his cheeky chops.

'So, you're the culprit,' I laughed, scooping him up.

I never told Sister Nivern who was responsible for her missing sandwich. Instead I asked Pearl to make an extra one for Richie until he went home.

20

There was a week to go before Christmas and Mrs Fry was recovering well from the overdose and miscarriage, but I worried about the boys going home and getting ill, and their mother doing something drastic. I'd learnt depression just didn't go away. Before my shift started I popped up to see Mrs Fry but she was sleeping and I didn't want to disturb her.

I heard a voice behind me say, 'She's stronger than you think, Hill. Mrs Fry's going home today.' It was Sister Steadman, the departmental sister.

'So are the boys,' I told her. 'I can't bear to think of them going back to that horrid house. They'll never get better there.'

Sister Steadman invited me into her office for a cup of tea and a chat. I told her about Mrs Fry's and Mrs Edwards's home, how the boys would never recover from the bronchitis while they lived there and how I was determined to go and see the Lady Almoner to ask her to do something.

Sister Steadman listened patiently and smiled. As she poured me a second cup she said, 'Hill, you must know there is a hierarchy at work here. You, I am afraid, are too far down the pecking order to be making demands of anyone. Housing isn't a matter for the hospital, you see; it is the local authority's responsibility, not the NHS.'

'But Sister ...'

She held her hand up to silence me; I sat back down in my seat and drank my tea to hush my tongue.

'What you need, Hill, is an ally who has influence with the Lady Almoner and the local authority. What you need is Miss Knox.'

'Miss Knox?' Who was this magical person?

'Miss Knox is a very old friend of the Lady Almoner's and mine. She is a health visitor on the district.'

'What's a health visitor?' I asked.

'That's a very good question,' smiled Sister. 'In our case she is our best chance at getting a referral to the local authority for a home to save those boys' lives. She is one of us, Hill. Miss Knox is a nurse, a very highly trained nurse who works in the community, specialising in the health care of infants and their families in their own homes.'

'Would you ring her and ask her to help, please, Sister?'

'I will telephone Miss Knox as soon as you vacate my office, Nurse Hill,' Sister told me. I jumped out of my seat and rushed back to Infants Ward to find Appleton and tell her there was hope.

★   ★   ★

It was with a heavy heart I got Georgie and Bobbie ready to be discharged that afternoon. Their breathing had stabilised, but for how long was the unasked question on everybody's lips. I prayed Sister Steadman was true to her word and would contact Miss Knox to ask if there was something she could do for the family. The boys were due to be discharged at two o'clock, but at four in the afternoon there was still no sign of either Mrs Fry or Mrs Edwards.

Sister Nivern bustled in to see what the delay was. 'Nurse Hill, are those boys still here?' she barked. 'Are the whole family planning on taking up residency in the hospital?'

'Their mothers haven't arrived yet, Sister.'

'Why does that not surprise me, given their most recent behaviour? If they think the State is going to pick up the bill for the care of their children they've got another think coming,' said Sister Skinflint accusingly.

'I'm sure they'll be here soon, Sister,' I replied, as I started to wonder if I should put the children back into their pyjamas and into bed. Surely they wouldn't abandon them and make them wards of the State? Maybe they thought it was the cousins' best chance of survival?

I read Georgie and Bobbie a story very badly; the whole time my eyes were on the clock. My shift had finished but I didn't want to just leave them. Sister would probably call the police if their mothers didn't come by bedtime, but I was due to meet my dad. I selfishly thought about how much I was looking forward to seeing him and having our lovely dinner at The Dorchester. Sarah, I told myself off sharply, you're feeling sorry for yourself for missing out on a posh dinner with your dad, while these fatherless boys don't even have a proper home to go to. I decided that I would just have to telephone the hotel and cancel. I couldn't leave Georgie and Bobbie to the authorities, I just couldn't.

At 4.15 pm I still hadn't done anything. Sister came back.

'Nurse Hill, you're off duty now. What are you still doing here?' she snapped, slightly triumphantly I thought.

I opened my mouth to find the words, and then I saw Mrs Edwards and Mrs Fry tearing down the corridor. A middle-aged lady in a royal blue winter coat followed behind them at a more dignified pace. Each mother bounded into the room and scooped up her boy and hugged them tightly to her chest.

'Better late than never, I suppose,' said Sister.

The lady in the royal blue coat followed them into the bay. Her hair was short in a pixie-like bob, shiny black and greying at the edges. She had a pair of glasses perched on the top of her head and wore large rose-coloured glass beads in three rings around her pinkish, slender throat. She was tall and slim and I could see the hem of her charcoal pencil skirt under her coat, which tapered off to a pair of long legs clad in sensible but elegant black leather shoes.

'We're getting a new flat. A spanking new council flat that no one's ever lived in before!' cried Mrs Fry.

'Thanks to Miss Knox,' said Mrs Edwards as she grinned at the lady in the royal blue coat.

'I'm only sorry I hadn't met you all before,' said Miss Knox softly. Sister Nivern's lip curled. She was the only one in the room who wasn't utterly delighted.

Miss Knox took in old Skinflint and said to her in a low though perfectly audible whisper, 'Sister, I have a favour to ask of you. The new flat will be ready next week, just in time for Christmas. Might little Georgie and Bobbie have a bed here until then? I'd hate anything serious to happen to them as a result of being sent home *yet again* to unsuitable living conditions. Is it in your power to grant them sanctuary?'

'See to it, Nurse,' agreed Sister begrudgingly, as she bustled off to take refuge in her office away from busybody do-gooders, hell bent on helping people who didn't deserve it.

'How did you do it?' I asked Miss Knox, wide-eyed.

'Hill, is it?' she asked me. I nodded. 'Why don't you come out with me on your community practice and let me show you how it's done?' she said playfully. 'Now, I'll leave you all to your celebrations,' and then she was gone.

I looked at the clock. It was 4.20 pm. If I got changed rapidly and ran for the bus I could still make dinner with Dad.

That evening I was filled with hope. I rode on the top deck of a London bus en route to see my dad for dinner brimming with Christmas cheer. I watched the lights of the big houses overlooking Hyde Park twinkle in the evening sky, and there was just a hint of frost settling on the footpaths, the grass and park benches. Everything was crisp and sparkling with the glow of the street lamps, the rustling of the last of the fallen leaves and the hot chestnut sellers at Speakers' Corner. A group of young friends were sprawled over the seats in front me – they were clearly not from London. They *Ooh*'d and *Ahh*'d at all the sights and got Wellington's Arch mixed up with Marble Arch. When the conductor announced the stop 'The Dorchester Hotel', I got up and heard one of the girls say, 'Look at the cars outside The Dorchester. No one goes there on the bus.' I smiled to myself as not only was I arriving by bus, but my favourite conductor Clifford had let me ride for free.

I passed through the revolving doors and into the lobby of The Dorchester Hotel. It was like entering another world – the cares of everyday life just slipped away. I almost bumped into the huge Christmas tree and gingerbread house that towered over the lobby and gallery. Everywhere was adorned with strings of baubles and greenery. In the distance, at the end of the long promenade, a choir of boys was gathered round a black grand piano singing Christmas carols. I tried to walk with as much dignity as I possibly could. I'd worn the black maxi dress with large floating sleeves from Biba and the snakeskin shoes I'd found the tenner in from Dad. Heads turned as everyone tried to figure out if I was somebody, and I, of course, was a nobody.

I spied Dad's familiar receding hairline over the top of *The Times* as he sat on one of a pair of richly upholstered side chairs engrossed in his newspaper, his long legs and big feet stretched out in front of him. I found it surprisingly comforting and reassuring to see him squeezed into the chair in his smart, well-cut tailored suit, stiff white shirt, tie and shiny black shoes; all handmade and beautiful and so Dad. I stood in front of him but he didn't notice me at first, then I gave a little cough and he lowered his paper, revealing thick black horn-rimmed spectacles sitting comfortably on a largish nose and ears. My father had been a boxer at university and a bomb disposal officer in the war; he definitely had received and given a punch or two. A man who'd served in India and worked in Iraq – he'd seen things and toiled for everything we had. His smile grew as he took me in.

'You've grown up,' he said, his voice deep and measured as always. 'Calls for a proper grown-up drink,' and he nodded to the waiter to come over.

I smiled back and sat down in the side chair opposite him. 'Hello, Dad.'

A little thrill of excitement rushed through me. The pleasure of the new dress, dinner at The Dorchester, being a grown up, but most of all an evening with my dad – just him and me. No brothers and sisters, no pets, no Mum and no business associates and telephone calls, just the two of us.

The waiter was already with us, poised to take our order. 'Good afternoon, Sir, Madam; how are you today?' he said, swiftly giving my dad and me a menu each.

'Very well, thank you,' replied my father. I smiled.

'We are still serving our speciality Christmas afternoon tea and we have a range of delicious early evening appetisers to choose from until the restaurant opens at six o'clock.'

'I get enough tea at home,' said my dad. 'We are booked into the restaurant at seven o'clock; I just want something to stave off starvation before we go through.'

He couldn't be doing with finger sandwiches and patisserie; he had an enormous appetite – we'd be having a minimum of three courses tonight with all the wines to match, at least.

'May I recommend the *smörgåsbord*,' said the affable waiter. 'There is a choice of two dishes per serving. You can select from beef, shrimp, herring, crabmeat, salami and cheese.'

'We'll have everything,' said my father, definitively shutting his menu. 'And two champagne cocktails as well.'

'Excellent choice, Sir,' responded the waiter, taking both our menus.

'Oh, and can you make them pink champagne. I do prefer pink champagne, don't you, Sarah?'

'Yes, Dad,' I grinned.

'Of course, Sir,' said the waiter, giving us a smile and a nod, then dashing off.

'Always rely on The Dorchester for a good meal,' said Dad. 'Mind you, I put my shoes outside my door for cleaning last night and no one picked them up.'

'Oh, dear. They look shiny enough,' I commented, looking down at his ever-so-highly-polished black Oxford shoes.

'They should be. When I saw they'd not been done this morning I cleaned them myself on the bath towels.' He chuckled. I laughed – that was so Dad.

'What you reading about?' I asked.

'The Royal Family's preparations for Christmas following Her Majesty's and the Duke of Edinburgh's return from Afghanistan visiting ...' and he glanced at the paper for the name of a faraway monarch, '... King Zahir Shah. Dangerous place, Afghanistan,' he said, now with a faraway look of concern.

I scowled a little; my family hadn't been half as keen on the Royal Family before the Queen came to open the hydro-electric plant Dad built in Scotland. My father had been rather taken with Elizabeth II, and there were rumours he was up for a knighthood.

'I just bought a new colour television for the sitting room,' Dad told me enthusiastically. 'We'll be able to watch the Queen's Speech in colour on Christmas Day. You are coming home for Christmas, aren't you?'

'No, Dad, I'm not. I'm on duty all through Christmas and the new year.'

'That's outrageous. They can't expect you to miss out on Christmas with your family.'

'They can and they do. And I want to. I want to be there; it's very hard for our patients and their families to be in hospital at Christmas. People still get sick no matter what day it is. And besides, I'm helping to organise the staff Christmas show.'

'Quite right. Don't want to let the side down,' he said gruffly, but then he gave me a big grin as the waiter brought over our pink champagne cocktails. 'Let's toast, to my daughter the nurse.'

'Almost a nurse,' I said, and my stomach flipped at the thought of my upcoming community practice and next set of exams.

'You've passed with flying colours so far.'

'Yes, but it's getting harder and harder. There's only a handful of us left now; they've either failed or dropped out.'

'Quite right – sorts the wheat out from the chaff.' He took another large sip and ordered us two more cocktails as our delicious-looking *smörgåsbord* arrived. He popped some shrimp into his mouth and I nibbled on a bit of cheese. 'Truth be told, your mother and I never realised you were so blessed in the brains department.'

Thanks Dad! I thought sulkily, but he wasn't telling me anything I didn't already know.

'I'm very proud of you, but now I see you could do even better. Why not transfer to do medicine at a well-respected hospital? I'd be happy, more than happy, to pay for everything, and you'd be a doctor, a well-paid, well-respected doctor. You could be so much more than a nurse.'

'No, Dad. Nursing is my calling. I want to be where I am needed, and I'm needed here,' I told him firmly.

He held his hands up in defeat, but I knew this wouldn't be the last time my parents would try and persuade me to switch careers; they were both fighters, but as I was discovering in Hackney, so was I.

21

Appleton and I had rows of silver tinsel wrapped round our necks and pins in our mouths as we dressed the children's choir. We'd spent the past fortnight making tinsel halos and cardboard candles with them. Some of the older children had made wings, which we'd pinned onto their backs, others had a cardboard lantern, and a very few of them had even made themselves pixie ears. It was a fairytale Christmas assortment.

'Are they supposed to be angels, a choir, fairies, elves or what?' said Andrews the Casualty Charge Nurse as he put his hand on his hip and pouted.

'Does it matter?' said Appleton, as she got up from the floor of the backstage area of the hospital's communal hall and stood back to admire the children's costumes. 'They look fantastic.'

'And how do I look?' said Andrews, sweeping back with a flourish for us to admire his ensemble.

Usually a picture of strength and calmness in his nurse's tunic, tonight Andrews was dressed in a tight-fitting black satin corseted dress with a long swaggered skirt and bustle.

241

His silhouette was topped with a huge black-and-white hat decked with plumes of feathers, ivy and tinsel. He gave a little wiggle and lifted his comedy bust saucily, fluttering his thick fake eyelashes.

'And just who are you supposed to be?' teased Appleton.

'The Queen of the Music Halls, Miss Marie Lloyd,' he said, blowing a kiss from his ruby red lips and singing the first line of 'The Boy I Love Is up in the Gallery.'

'I'll bet he is,' smirked Appleton. 'Very festive.'

'You're just jealous,' teased Andrews. 'Now, duckies, it's time to take your seats and leave us artistes to do the real work,' he said, ushering us away.

'But the children …'

'The children will be fine, won't you, kids?' They all gave a little cheer to confirm this. 'You two enjoy the show. You've earned it, and you wouldn't want to miss my performance, would you?'

Appleton and I did as we were told and went into the communal hall. We'd been working all week putting up the garlands we'd made with the children. We must have linked thousands of paper chains and covered a hundred stars in glitter, but it all looked so beautiful. The hall sparkled with their creations and the room was packed out with patients and staff eager to see the Christmas show. At the edge of the stage stood a huge Christmas tree glittering with fairy lights, and sitting next to it very primly was Maddox at an upright piano, ready to accompany the performers.

'Where are we going to sit?' I asked Appleton.

'I think we're going to have to stand at the back,' she said glumly.

We started to edge our way through the crowd but then I saw Lynch waving madly, indicating two empty seats next to her. Gratefully we crept along the crowded rows until we were seated in the middle of the third row next to Lynch.

'I've had a right job keeping these seats for you,' Lynch hissed as she shot a dirty look at a nurse behind who'd tutted as we'd sat down. 'But if people who've actually helped to put on the show don't get to see it, it's hardly the Christmas spirit, is it?' she said loudly.

Appleton and I grinned; good old Lynch. The red curtain started to lift and a hush fell in the hall. Maddox began banging away on the ivories and the hospital choir came on doing high kicks in a chorus line dressed as elves, singing, 'Another opening, another show, in Hackney, Dalston and Walthamstow.' When they'd finished Dr Holmes came on in black tie to act as Master of Ceremonies and introduced the next act – one of the hospital porters on the banjo. He plucked the strings with little skill and made a terrible din as he sang, 'I'm leaning on a lamp-post at the corner of the street, in case a certain little lady comes by,' completely unaware of the effect he was having on the audience as they winced and covered their ears. Lynch, Appleton and I shook with suppressed laughter as he sang. When he'd finished he got up to go and Lynch cried, 'Encore, encore,' and we

joined in with her. He sang it again; I guess he hadn't prac-
tised another song, and this time I think it was even worse.
The audience members around us shot us filthy looks as
they had to endure another rendition of the song and we
three girls rocked with laughter, tears rolling down our
faces.

Next was our tutor from Nurses' School, Sister Powell,
dressed in a green gown with flowers and butterflies pinned
all over it. She sang, 'She Sits Among the Cabbages and
Peas'. Huge peals of laughter rang out throughout the hall
and I looked down our row to see the only sour face in the
room belonged to her rival, Sister Connors. She was quickly
followed on by our very own Wade. She was dressed in a
long brown shirt, black hat and shawl and blouse, which I
was surprised at, and she was carrying a birdcage. Suddenly
a chorus of hospital porters joined her and she started singing 'My Old Man Said Follow the Van', hitching up her skirts
and kicking her legs as she pranced about the stage.

'You've got to hand it to her, she really is very good,'
whispered Lynch. 'But don't you ever tell her I said so.'

Wade had everyone on their feet clapping and cheering.
Audience members who were standing in the aisles and at
the back started linking arms and dancing round. One or
two well-trained porters even threw flowers on at Wade's
feet as she finished. She shone, her eyes sparkling, her skin
rosy with energy and excitement. 'Give us another one!'
shouted the usually shy Dr Guy Fleming, who was only a
few seats away from us.

'For you, Doctor, anything,' said Wade saucily as she tossed off her hat and shawl to let down her long curly chestnut hair. She really did look very pretty.

'She was born in the wrong century,' whispered Appleton in surprised awe.

Wade made her way through the doctors in the audience, sitting on laps and stroking cheeks, singing, 'She's my lady love, she is my dove'. As she wrapped her arms around Dr Guy's neck and planted him a kiss on the cheek he went as red as a beetroot with embarrassment. I saw's Lynch's hands balled into fists in her lap. 'She always has to take it too far,' she hissed.

Top of the bill was Andrews. He sauntered onto the stage with a cane in his hand, and drummed the stage for silence and attention. He took his time, drinking in the audience, allowing us to take him in too as he put one hand on his hip and turned sideways on so we could admire his trim profile.

'Is everybody happy?' he called out to the audience. There was an affirmative titter. 'I said, is everybody happy?' A huge cheer went up. 'Now you may have noticed we've been celebrating the unique musical talent of one of Hackney's finest, the Queen of Music Hall, Marie Lloyd. And tonight you lucky, lucky people are joined by the image of Marie herself, if not a little bit prettier, in the shape of yours truly. So ladies and gents I want you to take a deep breath and join in, because I know you all know the words, and if I see any miserable so and so not joining in, well – they'll have the pleasure of my very special attention,' and he began to sing and we all joined on the chorus.

I'm a young girl, and have just come over,
Over from the country where they do things big,
And amongst the boys I've got a lover,
And since I've got a lover, why I don't care a fig.

The boy I love is up in the gallery,
The boy I love is looking now at me,
There he is, can't you see, waving his handkerchief,
As merry as a robin that sings on a tree.

Everyone was singing, clapping and stamping their feet, and as Andrews finished his big number on came the children's choir, accompanied by Daniels dressed as a huge silver crescent moon. Very softly Andrews started to lead the children in 'By the Light of the Silvery Moon'. Those who could got to their feet and we all linked arms and swayed and sang along; our voices grew louder and louder until our song must have been heard all over the hospital. Lynch, Appleton and I belted out, 'I want to spoon, to my honey I'll croon love's tune,' with great gusto.

When the show was over, Appleton and I gave the infants supper and tucked them into bed, flecks of tinsel in their hair, and I swear each precious soul fell asleep with a smile on their lips. When we were sure everyone was asleep, we tiptoed to each of their beds and filled one of their socks with an orange, sweets and a sugar mouse, all bought and paid for by Sister Skinflint.

'She does have a heart after all,' whispered Appleton.

'I know, just for tonight we'll call her Sister Santa Claus,' I giggled.

Appleton and I linked arms and headed out of Infants Ward to join our friends at the Adam & Eve, and then get a few hours sleep before we were due back for Christmas morning. I wouldn't have missed it for the world. It was one of the happiest Christmases of my life.

22

March 1972, and it was the usual early morning skirmish: Maddox hogging the shower so there wasn't enough hot water for everyone, Lynch oversleeping and then unable to find the studs for her collar, but unusually I was in mufti, ready for my first day of community practice. Nervously nibbling down toast and forcing down my morning tea, I hovered by the kitchen sink in a bright yellow ribbed turtleneck jumper with matching knee-high socks and black flat pumps. My skirt had triangles of bright yellow patches too, mixed in with browns and oranges. My hair was down and loose rather than in a tight bun, and I even wore a touch of lipstick and mascara on a working day; it was nice to be out of uniform, to be an individual for a change.

The bell was ringing again. 'If that's another one of Miss Valance's so-called gentleman callers, tell them we're being watched by the Vice Squad,' shouted Lynch.

I stuck my head out of the window, but it wasn't a man, it was Wade. She had a small brown suitcase with her – oh no, this couldn't be good.

I let her in. She looked like she'd been up half the night, her hair was a mess and her eyes were smudged and puffy.

'The long and the short of it is – Home Sister's turfed me out. Can I stay here?' asked Wade as she poured herself a cup of tea and helped herself to my toast.

'Why have you been thrown out?' asked Lynch suspiciously as she rapidly brushed her dark hair out and pinned it.

'She's just a bitter, bitter woman,' answered Wade.

Lynch and Maddox both scowled. Wade had caught us on the hop and she knew it; none of us had the time to get to the bottom of what had happened.

'I'm going to be late. I've got to get to the clinic,' I said as I picked up my brown leather school satchel. 'You can stay but it's just temporary.'

Wade smiled and flopped down onto the sofa. 'It's my day off and I need to catch up on my beauty sleep. Shall I sleep here or take your bed, Hill?'

I picked up some blankets and pillows and dropped them into her lap.

'There you go, now I've really got to get going.'

Maddox and Lynch nodded and quickly picked up handbags and coats too as we all headed out of our flat for work.

'I don't want her getting too comfortable,' said Lynch.

'Or she'll never go,' added Maddox.

'I'm sure she won't be any trouble,' I lied. We raced for the bus after being delayed by our uninvited guest.

Without even looking up from her paperwork the uppity receptionist told me, 'The health visitors' room is on the right at the top of the stairs.' I took a deep breath and walked up. The office was lined with eight heavy wooden desks. Each was its own little oasis with a filing cabinet, wastepaper basket and chair, and plenty of space between. There was a little cubbyhole of an office in the corner belonging to the health visitors' clerk, who sat at a large typewriter. Her fingers were heavy on the keys and the strike of the ribbon created a clattering sound that mixed in with the ring of a telephone. A resounding ding filled the room as she came to the end of a line and then she pulled the lever to start again. Some of the desks were as neat as a new pin, others were scattered with papers, coffee cups and even a half-eaten, curled-up ham sandwich.

Miss Knox was on the telephone, seated at a desk with a dark green blotter, pen, mug, ink pot and letter rack – all her papers were neatly stacked in a wicker tray. She had a small silver fountain pen in her hand and was making notes in a purple diary as she listened to her caller and nodded responsively. She noticed me and gave a little wave, then her attention was drawn away again, her head cocked to one side. Her chair was pushed back from the desk and I was surprised to see so much leg. She was wearing a mini dress with a large collar and a large silver cuff bracelet at her wrist. A long single row of large red beads hung loosely round her neck. Clearly this is a woman who loves fashion and knows how to make the most of herself, I couldn't help but think admiringly.

It was just me, Miss Knox and the clerk in the office so far, and I didn't know if I should sit or stand. I didn't want to sit at someone else's desk in case they turned up but there were no spare chairs, and equally I didn't want to hover and listen in to what might be a confidential conversation. Miss Knox saw my dilemma and mouthed to me to make us both a cup of coffee. I gratefully scuttled off to find the kitchen and returned with black coffee in two white cups with saucers, a little milk jug and sugar bowl with tongs, all neatly presented on a wooden tray.

Miss Knox was just finishing her call. 'It's not a problem at all, I will be with you within the hour. I have a student nurse with me – would you prefer me to come on my own?' God, why would anybody let me in their home? I said to myself, suddenly unsure whether I'd get any experience at all on my week in the district. 'Well, that's very kind of you, Mrs Gould. Nurse Hill and I will look forward to seeing you soon.'

Miss Knox looked appreciatively at the tray and picked up the milk jug and added a little milk to her coffee.

'I'm so glad you picked the nicest cups. I do think the better the cup the better the taste,' she smiled as she took a little sip. 'Delicious. After this I'll make some tea. I always say you need a cup of tea after a cup of coffee.'

* * *

Miss Knox threw her scales and bag onto the back seat of her red mini, slipped elegantly in and turned on the ignition. 'Get in, Sarah.'

She twiddled the knobs on the radio until the Rolling Stones' 'Honky Tonk Woman' was blaring out at us. 'Personally I think Mick Jagger is a bit of a big-headed lout,' she told me as she put on her seatbelt and we headed off. 'One of my friends was at school with him and he was always telling anyone that had ears he was going to be famous. You can't deny it, though, it's good music.'

It was warm for early spring and Miss Knox wound the windows down as we drove so she could wave and say hello to the mothers pushing their prams along. I was surprised to see so many people smiling and waving at her. We stopped at a traffic light and a man pulled up on his bike.

'Good morning, Miss Knox,' he said cheerfully. 'How you keeping?'

'All's well, thank you, Mr Parker. How's your wife and that lovely bonny baby?'

'They're both fine and dandy, thank you,' he grinned.

'Well, I'm glad to hear it. I'm glad my lights are on too.'

'Yes. Heath gave in, in the end.'

'Well done. You deserve it,' she grinned as the traffic lights changed and we drove off. I could still see Mr Parker giving a little wave in the wing mirror.

'They're a lovely family. Not easy having a new baby in the middle of a strike, but they stuck together and now they're much better off for it.'

'What strike?' I asked.

'Did you not notice your lights not working, Sarah?' she asked, raising an eyebrow. 'Seven weeks Mr Parker and his colleagues at Hackney Power Station were on strike.'

'Oh, yes, of course,' I said, feeling a bit silly – I hadn't made the connection.

'I bet his wife's glad to see him back to work.'

'Yes, it must be very hard with the money not coming in,' I sympathised.

'Yes, and it's not easy suddenly having your husband under your feet all day either,' Miss Knox joked.

We pulled up outside Mrs Gould's high-rise block of flats. I looked up at the twenty-storey block; it was mass of vertical and criss-crossed lines that put together made up the uniform bricks, windows, doors and balconies of the tower. Its solid, relentless shape was only broken by the different shades of grey squares that represented each home.

'We've got four newborn visits to do before lunchtime, Sarah,' explained Miss Knox. 'What Mrs Gould needs is a friendly ear. Now do respond and be your charming self if she talks to you, but remember I'm here to listen and that means you're here to observe and do a bit of washing up and help with the children while we talk.'

We waited in the lobby for the lift. Miss Knox pressed the button repeatedly but nothing happened.

'It's broken again,' she tutted. 'Glad to see you've got your sensible shoes on, Sarah – it's eighteen flights to Mrs Gould's flat.'

The door behind us opened and I heard a baby's cry. A woman with short mahogany brown hair stood in the doorway, a baby against her chest, a toddler holding one hand, another holding the edge of her brown belted dress.

'Oh Miss Knox,' the woman cried. 'I went to the get the baby's milk from the clinic but the baby's only gone and soiled himself halfway there. He's screaming hungry but I couldn't take him in like that. Those receptionists give me filthy looks as it is.'

'Don't worry, Mrs Gould, I've got some milk in the car you can have,' soothed Miss Knox. 'Why don't you take the baby up to the flat and then Nurse Hill and I will bring up Beth and Josie with us.'

'Thank you. I've had a fortnight of climbing up and down those bloody stairs. I have to cart down the pram with the baby in it. God knows that's an accident waiting to happen – my heart's in my throat the whole time and I'm worried sick that something will happen to Josie and Beth, left up in the flat on their own. I have to run back up again to get them and bring them down all those steps and they both always want to be carried. Then it's the same when I get home, only then I've got the shopping as well. It's a nightmare, a total bloody nightmare.'

'It's not good enough, Mrs Gould. I will ring the council as soon as I get back to the clinic and tell them to get a repair team here,' said Miss Knox, taking hold of the children's hands as their mother wearily started to make her way up the stairs.

* * *

Miss Knox sent me straight into the kitchen with Josie and Beth and the NHS dried milk for the baby. The noise level was deafening; in this tiny space the wailing of one baby and the whining of two toddlers seemed so much louder than the whole of Infants Ward – there was no escaping it. I peeked through at Miss Knox and Mrs Gould on the sofa as the mother tried to soothe the crying babe, but nothing was going to put a stop to his wailing but a bottle of milk. I put on the kettle as instructed to make Mrs Gould a much-needed cup of tea and got out some beakers from the cupboard for the toddlers to stack and play tea parties with on the kitchen table. I knew from Infants Ward that the baby's bottle needed to be sterilised but there was no big steriliser here like in the milk kitchen. I washed up a battered old pan in the crowded sink and planned to wash the rest of it as soon as the baby was settled. I boiled the bottle and the teat in the saucepan of bubbling water and then made up the feed as quickly as I could, cooling it down in a bowl full of cold water before practically running into the sitting room with it. While that baby was howling it felt like every second was a minute and every minute was an hour – I really felt for poor Mrs Gould.

The baby practically grabbed the bottle out of my hands and started sucking, and calmness fell upon the flat. I brought through the tea for Miss Knox and Mrs Gould and then went back to the kitchen to watch Josie and Beth. As I stood at the sink doing the dishes I couldn't help but hear Mrs Gould and Miss Knox talking.

'He comes home, eats his dinner and barely says a word to me or the kids. Has a wash and a change of shirt and then he's off out again until the small hours. Gambling and chasing women. I have to keep the rent book, my housekeeping and family allowance at my mum's or he'd have it off me,' she explained. The baby had fallen asleep with the empty bottle still clenched between his gums. Mrs Gould plucked it from his lips and put him down for a nap in the battered old pram I'd hauled up the eighteen flights of stairs for her. 'We're always short, Miss Knox, and it's not him who suffers, it's us – there's nothing in my purse but a few coppers. He's off living the single life while me and the kids are hiding behind the sofa when the rent man comes.' She collapsed into Miss Knox's arms, weeping.

I poured a glass of milk for Josie and Beth and sat down at the kitchen table with them. Miss Knox waited until Mrs Gould had recovered herself and then said gently, 'I'm going to make a few phone calls when I get back to the office. What would be the biggest help to you and the children?'

'If the lift worked it would mean I didn't have to use up every scrap of energy I've got left just getting them in and out of the flat. I know I'm a bit short-tempered with Josie and Beth but they're always pulling at my hair and my skirt, wanting to be picked up all the time when I'm trying to sort the baby out. I've only got one pair of hands. I barely have time to comb my hair and brush my teeth. I'm tired to the bone, Miss Knox. I'm doing my best, I really am, but it's just never good enough. I'm a bad mother, aren't I?' she asked pitifully.

'Anyone would find it tough in your circumstances, Mrs Gould. You are not a bad mother, you are a good mother and you deserve a break and a little bit of help. How would you feel about Josie and Beth starting nursery? You could have a little more time for you and the baby, and they could burn off some of that energy learning new things and playing with lots of new toys.'

'I'd love it but I haven't got the money for it, and what would the nursery think of me? I do my best to keep them neat but they need new shoes and clothes. I've only ever had a few things and they've been washed so many times it's all practically threadbare. Especially the baby's things; they've already done both my girls and my sister's four children and I think she got them off our cousin in Hammersmith.'

As we drove away in Miss Knox's mini to our next visit I was amazed at what I'd seen. I'd been wondering why anyone would even let a health visitor through the front door – surely mums were busy enough with babies and small children and would resent some busybody nurse checking up on them. But now I realised she was both needed and wanted.

When we got back to the office for a quick break before the afternoon's baby clinic Miss Knox sprang into action. I heard her tell somebody at the council that if anything happened to Mrs Gould or anyone else in the flats as a result of their negligence they were liable. She listened and then said rather smoothly, 'Well, tomorrow would be acceptable but this afternoon would be tremendous.' She smiled and nodded that her request had been met. 'Thank you. I'll be visiting the tower block again later this week and will be very glad to use the lift and not the stairs. Goodbye.'

I was so impressed with the polite but firm way she talked to people to get the best for her families. Next Miss Knox rung a trust fund to get the money for a nursery place for Beth and a play school place for Josie, and money for new shoes and clothes for all three children. She then popped downstairs to see the GP and asked him to see Mrs Gould as she was worried she was suffering from post-natal depression. I couldn't believe she was making such a difference and I thought about all the times I'd wished I could help my patients. Here was a way you could do it. Not just treating illness but helping to prevent it. By lunchtime my mind was made up: I was going to be a health visitor one day.

The baby clinic was at the church hall. We'd barely got the doors open before mothers, babies and small children descended upon us. Fortunately they left the prams outside in the sun, as about forty mothers and three times as many children came and went during the two-hour clinic. Miss Knox kept me busy with helping the clerk to find the records for each child, keeping the place clean, wiping the scales when one of the children had a little accident and setting up a play corner to keep the older children amused. I loved chatting to the mums while they waited for Miss Knox. I played with the children and cooed over a never-ending stream of gorgeous little babies. I couldn't give any advice, after all what did I know, but I felt I was helping in some small way by listening and lending a hand. They all came away smiling. How Miss Knox managed to see all those women in such a short space of time was a mystery to me then.

'We all love Miss Knox,' one mum told me. 'Some of the other health visitors are right snooty mares and think they know it all, but not Miss Knox. You could never tell she didn't have kids of her own, she's got such a way with babies.'

A sudden thought entered my head – do health visitors not have babies either? Was it the same as for Sister or Matron, a life spent of caring for other people's children and never your own? No, I was sure some of the health visitors at the clinic were married women with grown-up children. Good. But I realised they must have given up nursing when they had a family and started health visiting once their child-bearing years had ended. I didn't want to wait that long, I didn't want to give up my career, my vocation – but I didn't want to miss out on being a mother either. Was it possible to have both? And my mind raced back to the Women's Lib meetings I'd been going to with Maddox – I wanted an answer; I wanted a choice.

We returned to the clinic at four o'clock and Miss Knox sent me home for the day, saying, 'You go home now, Sarah, it's just paperwork for me. And well done, it was good to have you on the team today.'

I left with such a smile on my face and sailed all the way to the bus stop. After such a busy day, seeing so many people, it was good to sit back on the top deck of a red bus and just let the day's events wash over me. It was true, visiting people at home and in their communities didn't have the same level of dramatic excitement as hospital life, but seeing them in their own environments with the people who touched their lives gave the work a level of insight that wasn't possible on a ward. I felt that just watching Miss Knox and listening to the mothers was teaching me something I'd never learn in the classroom. This was real life; the rules were different here. Seeing people at home provided a window into their lives – you weren't just one of many nurses coming and going, you were their health visitor, you had a responsibility to them.

I thought about the drive back to the clinic in Miss Knox's car, and the way she'd spoken about the mums and the challenges they faced with such respect and understanding.

'The day you go in and think you know it all, Sarah, is the day you make a terrible mistake,' she told me. 'The health visitor is the least important person in the room – you haven't gone to that house for them to listen to you, you've gone to listen to them. Everyone needs help and support when they have children; it's just what is needed most is different for each mother. If you don't know them, if they can't trust you – what help can you be to them? We are such a small part of their lives so we need to be an effective part; the day I can't be of some use to a mother is the day I pack this lark in.' She said this smiling, but she meant it.

Before my key was even in the lock of our little flat I could hear T. Rex's 'Get It On' at full blast on my Dansette. The door swung open to reveal Edie, rollers in her hair, smoking a cigarette and putting her bright red lipstick on, looking at her reflection in the kitchen window. She was wearing a pale pink négligée and her hips were swinging from side to side in time with the music. As she heard the door shut behind me she swung round in surprise.

I turned the music down. 'Wade, you'll get us thrown out too with all this racket,' I scolded her.

'Hill, you're home early,' she exclaimed without batting an eyelid. 'This health visiting malarkey is obviously a lot easier than nursing,' she chortled as she started to pull her rollers out one by one, letting down tight glossy chestnut curls. 'Anyway, I'm glad you're home early before Sour Puss and Iron Drawers get back from work because we, pet, are going out tonight. So, quick smart, get your glad rags on, the lads are picking us up at six o'clock.'

'What lads?'

'Eric and Ernie.'

I opened my mouth – she was not serious. I know she'd bragged about being on the stage on the Pier with Morecambe and Wise in their early career, but I thought it was all hot air.

'Don't be silly, pet, not them,' she laughed. 'Eric and Ernie Goldberg. Eric's a theatrical agent, mind, but Ernie's a cab driver. Still, he can give us all a lift can't he.'

I felt silly at feeling a little disappointed.

'Eric wants to discuss my comeback.'

'What comeback?'

'To the stage, to the boards, the footlights,' she explained, sweeping out both her arms and curtseying to her adoring crowd of fans.

'What's that got to do with me?'

'Double date. Ernie is Eric's younger brother. He's just set him up with a cab. Trying to keep him on the straight and narrow.'

'I'm not sure I want a blind double date with someone who needs keeping on the straight and narrow, thank you,' I replied primly.

'It's not drugs, or alcohol, or gambling, or sex. It's the saxophone.' I looked perplexed.

'He was in a band on Ernie's books,' Wade continued. 'But there's no money in that jazz music. Rock and roll is where it's at but he likes Bix Beiderbecke, for crying out loud.' Wade stepped into a long sleeveless empire red gown covered in black butterflies.

'You look lovely,' I told her admiringly.

Wade did a little twirl. 'Four pounds from Selfridges. It's called the irresistible flirt.'

'Figures,' I responded as I went to the bathroom to wash and get changed.

'Did I mention they're taking us to the Playboy Club?' she called.

There was no arguing with Wade, and you couldn't deny she knew how to have a good time. Besides, I was intrigued; a jazz-loving Jewish saxophone-playing cab driver – now that's got be interesting. But maybe we shouldn't mention to Maddox we'd been to the Playboy Club, I thought, as I patched up my make-up.

Ernie parked his cab in a side street. It was nice to have a chance to wear my Biba black maxi dress and be on Park Lane again. I looked fondly at the twinkling lights of The Dorchester as I walked under the canopy of the Playboy Club.

The doorman held open the door for our foursome. 'I'll hope you'll be lucky tonight, Mr Goldberg,' he said.

'I intend to be,' smirked Eric as he pinched Wade's bottom and she gave a little whoop of excitement.

I held back with Ernie. He scowled at his brother. 'Don't worry, Sarah, I'll buy us both tickets to the buffet and there's a free disco. Leave the gambling to those with more money than sense, shall we?' he suggested as he offered me his arm.

I took it. I only had three pounds for an emergency cab fare home in case I didn't like my date, and there was no way I was risking that on the roulette tables.

When we walked in I heard the same T. Rex track as Wade has been listening to back at the flat. There were Bunny Girls everywhere – carrying drinks, at the gambling tables, waiting on tables, and sitting at tables with men smoking large cigars and sipping champagne. A Bunny Girl showed us to the booth Eric had reserved. She was wearing a bright orange satin bodice with matching pert orange rabbit ears, a fluffy white tail, a white collar and black bow tie at the neck and white cuffs at the wrist. Ernie tipped her twenty pence and asked her to get us a bottle of bubbly.

'That's very generous of you,' said Wade.

'Not to worry, Edie. This is work – one way or another it'll be my client that pays for it,' he guffawed as he lit up a cigarette and passed the packet to Wade.

We each scanned the room, taking in the hedonistic scene. Ernie pointed at a man at the bar surrounded by Bunnies with a bald rounded head and prominent chin, a largish pointed nose and plump lips wearing a dinner jacket.

'Hey, isn't that Telly Savalas?' he said, nudging me.

I strained to see but I hadn't worn my glasses and it was all a little hazy.

'I'm going to have a look,' he said. 'And I'll get us some tickets for the buffet. Shall I get you his autograph if it is him?'

'No, don't,' I implored as the orange satin Bunny brought over our champagne.

I turned my back on Wade and Eric as they drank from each other's glass at the same time, and I was very relieved when Ernie came back.

'It is him,' he grinned.

'It's who?' snapped Eric.

'Telly Savalas,' said Ernie.

'Oh, maybe I should go and introduce myself,' said Eric, adjusting his bow tie, slicking back his brown hair and then dashing off, leaving Wade to her own devices.

'There's quite a crowd around him,' I said as I squinted at the fevered scene at the bar.

'I should think so. He's handing out ten pound notes.'

'He must be loaded!' shrieked Wade.

'I don't think he's caught up with decimalisation. He thinks they're the old brown ten bob notes. Every girl in the place is making a beeline for him.'

We laughed. 'Not just the girls, either,' said Wade, gesturing to the lurking figure of Eric trying to get through the crowd around the American star. 'I don't think your brother is going to make me a star any time soon,' Wade said wistfully to Ernie.

'Well, you've got too many legs for a start,' smirked Ernie.

'I beg your pardon?' said Wade, offended and confused.

'It's mainly dog acts on his books, animals for TV, film, ads, that sort of thing.'

'It's what?' shouted Wade. She took up the bottle of champagne and emptied it into our glasses, and called our waitress over to order another. 'Bring us three more bottles,' she told her.

'I like to see a dog pay for that,' she grinned.

* * *

I didn't want to have a hangover or be up too late so I only had another glass. By the time I snuck off Ernie was singing softly into Wade's ear and telling her the life stories of Duke Ellington and Bix Beiderbecke. Despite the age gap – he was twenty-six and she was forty-one – they seemed well matched. I was glad I'd brought the cab fare with me; there was no way I was getting into a car with champagne-fuelled Ernie behind the wheel. You had to hand it to Wade, though: that girl had plenty of bounce. She could give a twenty-something Playboy Bunny a run for their money any day of the week.

Miss Knox was flicking through her case notes to find the house number as we sat in her red mini outside a row of neat terraced houses.

'Aha, number 16,' she said triumphantly. 'Sarah, there are some leaflets in a box on breastfeeding on the back seat. Would you get one with all the language translations on, please. Dr Montgomery asked me to visit this Asian family with a first baby as the father came to see him and said the mother's struggling to breastfeed.'

I looked in the box and pulled out one of the leaflets. It was covered in so many languages – I hoped we'd be able to talk to her. I knew from the hospital it was very challenging when the patient didn't speak English, especially if they were in distress.

Miss Knox knocked on the dark green, freshly painted front door. A good-looking man in a long white tunic and grey trousers opened it.

'Can I help you?' he asked.

'Mr Ahmad?' Miss Knox enquired.

'Yes,' he answered.

'I'm Miss Knox, the health visitor, and this is my student, Nurse Hill. Dr Montgomery asked me to call,' she explained.

The man smiled. He had brilliant white straight teeth and full lips. His eyes were heavy lidded with thick black eyebrows and a mass of dark curly hair. He must have only been a few years older than me.

'Oh, thank you for coming, please do come in,' he said as we walked through the newly decorated hall into a smart neat living room. 'Do take a seat. My wife will be through with the baby in just a moment. Can I get you both a cup of tea?'

We both readily agreed and didn't have to wait long before a woman wearing a pale pink sari, with the longest rich black hair and huge brown almond-shaped eyes, came in holding a sleeping baby nestled in her shoulder. She smiled shyly and sat down opposite us.

'Hello, Mrs Ahmad,' said Miss Knox cheerfully. But she only got another shy smile in reply. Miss Knox picked up the leaflet on breastfeeding and gave it to the new mother. She asked her gently and slowly, 'Can you read any of these languages?'

The woman studied the leaflet for a few moments and then nodded.

Miss Knox smiled and then the woman started to read. 'A breastfeeding mother needs plenty of iron,' she read in English from the leaflet.

'I'm so sorry, I didn't realise you spoke English, Mrs Ahmad,' apologised Miss Knox. 'Dr Montgomery …'

'There is the root of the misunderstanding. Dr Montgomery persistently confuses me with another woman. Mrs Ahmad next door doesn't speak English, but Mrs Nazeera Begum does.' As per usual I was confused, but unusually Miss Knox looked puzzled too. 'It is my family's tradition for women to keep their names after they are married,' explained Mrs Begum. 'And I don't speak English very well; I do find the nuances most challenging,' she said with a wry smile.

Miss Knox threw back her head and hooted. Mr Ahmad brought in a tray with glass cups and saucers brimming with freshly brewed tea. It tasted sweet, a bit too sweet for me, but Miss Knox lapped it up.

'Delicious,' she said. 'How do you make this?'

'In a pan with creamy milk and sugar,' replied Mr Ahmad.

'I am sorry little Tarek is sleeping,' Mrs Begum apologised. 'We've had a sleepless night, all of us.'

'He's six weeks old now, isn't he?' began Miss Knox, popping over to look at the sleeping baby admiringly. 'Oh, isn't he beautiful.' She squeaked in delight as the baby's lips started twitching and sucking in his sleep.

'I think I've seen sunrise every morning since he was born,' yawned Mrs Begum.

'I see and what are his sleeping and feeding patterns like in the day?'

'He feeds fitfully. He thrashes about and beats me with his little fists and then when I do finally manage to get him on he feeds till I'm sore and then sleeps.'

'And how long does he sleep for?'

'He usually sleeps from ten o'clock till well after lunchtime. Feeds and then sleeps again. During the day apart from the soreness it's not too bad. I get to have a little nap and do some housework, but at night when he's not feeding he's crying. I think I must be doing something very wrong.'

'You sound very dedicated to me,' said Miss Knox. 'What do you think you'd like to change?'

'I'd like to get a few hours' continuous sleep. And all this stopping and starting is no good at all. I feel like a zombie walking around with my eyes half shut.'

'Well, we can discuss feeding techniques, and how you can treat and then prevent soreness, because that must be making you feel terribly low.'

'It is, it is,' said Mrs Begum tearfully. 'At home I would have my mother, sisters, aunts and cousins to help me, but here I have to do everything myself. Mushtaq runs a restaurant so he has to leave at five o'clock and isn't back till very late and he's been sleeping on the sofa so he can get some rest because he can't work if he's had no sleep too. But I feel very alone, especially at night. I miss my home and my family.'

The baby woke and started to cry too and Mr Ahmad rushed round to comfort his wife and child. Miss Knox offered to take the baby and started to stroke from the top of his nose downwards until he relaxed and stopped crying, and then she cradled him in her arms.

'We have only been in England for just over a year,' explained Mr Ahmad. 'Having the baby in a strange country without the support of family has been very hard for both of us, but especially my wife.'

'Where are your family, Mr Ahmad?' asked Miss Knox.

'What's left of them are in Bangladesh. I was studying at university in Dhaka when the war broke out at the beginning of last year. My wife and I both come from academic families and my family sent us immediately to England with suitcases full of the gold jewellery my mother wore to her wedding, and valuable cloth. The Pakistani militia had already started to round up and butcher members of the intelligentsia, but my parents did not want to abandon their country; they only wanted to keep their only child safe. Both my mother and father had been forced to flee from India to Dhaka when I was just a baby after Indian independence; they knew all too well what lay ahead. I hadn't finished my degree so I cannot enter into a university here. So, to my shame I sold my mother's gold and the cloth and bought a restaurant here in Hackney, and bought this house.'

'Mushtaq, your parents wanted you to sell it. That's why they sent it with us; not to keep it safe,' comforted Mrs Begum as she wiped away her tears.

Miss Knox waited for the couple to regain their composure. We talked a little more about Mr Ahmad's new business. He owned the Bengal Tiger and was surprised when I told him how much I loved curry.

'Do you? I keep finding people come in expecting bananas and raisins in their rice,' chortled Mr Ahmad.

'My father cooks curry. He served in India. He loves to boast of how he had a beautiful Indian girlfriend whom he took to the officers' mess, and one night a rather rude captain asked him what he was doing bringing in a native into civilised company or some such rubbish and, before my father could give him what for, the girl said, "Captain, my people were creating poetry, music and great buildings while your people were still living in damp caves."'

They all laughed and Mrs Begum brought in some glasses of water with homemade samosas that were delicious. Baby Tarek started to get a little fidgety again; his open mouth was rooting around for a feed.

'Do you think he's hungry?' asked Miss Knox.

'Yes,' said Mrs Begum.

'Would you like me to talk you through a feeding technique?'

'Please, Miss Knox.'

Miss Knox went and sat next to the mother and baby. 'Now I want you to get comfortable because you know feeding takes some time and the more relaxed you are the better.'

Mr Ahmad brought some extra cushions and put them under his wife's back.

'Now, when you are ready, Mrs Begum, I want you to bring the baby up from underneath the breast. Line him up nose to nipple and when you see him open that beautiful little mouth nice and wide, put him on with as much of the nipple in the mouth as you can. What you don't want is him sucking on the end as that will make you unnecessarily sore. Are you ready?'

Mrs Begum nodded. She followed Miss Knox's instructions as the health visitor gently guided her through it, and then the baby was on, sucking peacefully.

'Well done, Mrs Begum, that's perfect. How does that feel?' asked Miss Knox.

'It doesn't hurt. Oh, thank you, thank you, Miss Knox,' beamed Mrs Begum. She looked admiringly at her baby, his little fist wrapped around her finger as she fed.

Mr Ahmad looked thrilled and kissed his wife on the forehead. 'Well done, Nazeera,' he told her.

'Would now be a good time to talk a little more about feeding and sleeping patterns?' asked Miss Knox.

'Please,' they both said together.

'It may be we need to encourage Tarek to feed a little more regularly and sleep a little less in the day, so he sleeps a lot more and feeds much less at night.'

'That would be wonderful,' said Mrs Begum.

'When you are ready I want you to write out the usual pattern of your day and then we can discuss where you might want to add in a feed and if necessary what we can do to shorten Tarek's daytime naps,' explained Miss Knox, producing her lovely little fountain pen and notebook from her bag.

Miss Knox spent another half hour talking about what they could do. With each growing minute I could see how they knew something needed to shift a bit, that all the love and care was there, but they just needed an old hand like Miss Knox to give them some tips and advice that would work for their little family. After we'd been there an hour Miss Knox asked if there was anything else they'd like to discuss before we left. The couple exchanged a quick look.

'My husband knows some men who've recently arrived with their families from Bangladesh,' began Mrs Begum. 'The men work in a local factory and the owner said he would provide accommodation, but the flats he has given them aren't very nice. They are usually very shabby, without proper bathrooms and kitchens, and where two or three families have to share a flat meant for only one family.'

'I see,' answered Miss Knox thoughtfully.

'The women don't speak any English. One of your beautifully translated leaflets would be no good to them as they cannot read in their own language,' said Mrs Begum, casting her eyes to the floor.

'They are from villages,' explained Mr Ahmad. 'Life is very different there than in the cities.'

'Are the women and children often sick?' asked Miss Knox.

'Yes, very often,' replied Mrs Begum.

'Where are they?'

'Near Brick Lane,' answered Mr Ahmad.

'I'm afraid that's not my patch. But I could refer them.'

'I think they would hide if anyone called,' said Mrs Begum.

'Quite possibly,' Miss Knox said thoughtfully. 'What about coming to baby clinic?'

'A meeting of English-speaking women in a church hall – I am sorry to say I do not think they would go there either,' responded Mrs Begum.

I looked at Miss Knox, my eyes wide. I had an idea but I didn't want to overstep the mark. The health visitor noted my pleading eyes and asked me, 'Do you have a suggestion, Nurse Hill?'

'What about a mothers' group? Somewhere nearer Brick Lane that Mrs Begum could invite them to and we could get started with some tea and biscuits from the church. You could pop in now and again if Mrs Begum thought it was a good idea, and she could translate for you.'

'That sounds like an excellent idea to me. What do you say, Mrs Begum? A weekly Bangladeshi mothers' group?'

'Oh yes, please. I would love that, I would absolutely love it,' said the lovely, happy, smiling Mrs Begum.

As we were leaving Mr Ahmad asked us both if we would accept his invitation to dine in his restaurant with a group of our friends for free to say thank you. Once we were in the car Miss Knox told me, 'What a beautiful family. I cannot accept the invitation to eat *gratis* at Mr Ahmad's restaurant, of course – it would not be ethical. But why don't you take a group of your pals and enjoy yourself, Sarah. You did very well today.'

As she put her key in the ignition and started up the engine she turned those sparkling eyes on me and asked, 'Have you thought about becoming a health visitor one day, Sarah?'

23

I'd been working on the busiest department in the hospital, Casualty, under the watchful eye of Charge Nurse Andrews, for the weeks following my community practice. He took great delight in giving me as much practical experience as possible in the run up to my final year of practical and written exams. The first thing I did when I came on duty for the night shift was check the patient board to see who'd been admitted so far and where they were in their treatment. As I scanned the chart I could see Andrews out of the corner of my eye smirking at me.

'Still feeling a bit green about the gills, are we, Hill?' he teased.

The previous night Andrews had sent me to assist the surgeon performing an emergency operation in the small Casualty theatre. It was on a young man who'd smashed up his legs in a motorcycle accident. I hadn't yet worked as a theatre nurse and I couldn't help but feel queasy; it was a bit nerve-racking, and the surgeon cursed loudly the whole time as he worked. I was standing still under the hot theatre lights for so long I thought I would faint and end up impaling myself on the tray full of surgical instruments. Luckily I didn't pass out, but when I emerged from theatre Andrews took one look at my pale, drawn face and sent me to have a lie down and a cup of tea for ten minutes. I'd felt a bit silly, but the mix of heat, blood and lack of air as I stood in the same spot for three hours had taken its toll on me.

'Don't beat yourself up about it, Hill,' Andrews said, patting me on the back. 'You're the first student I've had all year who hasn't thrown up during her theatrical début.'

I jokingly huffed and turned my attention back to the patient board.

'It's a bit quiet tonight, Charge Nurse,' I remarked.

'I know – it's been like the morgue in here for the past hour. I've only got the one patient at the moment and that's one of the hospital porters who's done his back in. Still, let's make the most of it – get the kettle on and let's break open that nice tin of biccies I've been saving in the supply cupboard.'

Once I'd returned with the tea and biscuits, Andrews was looking irritated and flicking through a stack of forms.

'Have you seen this?' he asked, wafting the pieces of paper under my nose.

'No. What are they?'

'One of those new lah-di-dah hospital managers they've brought in who doesn't know a patient's arse from his elbow has sent down a list of instructions on how I should run my ward.'

'Really?' I said. I took one off him and looked at it. 'Someone gets paid to write this stuff?' I asked in disbelief.

'Talk about teaching your grandmother to suck eggs,' said Andrews as he aggressively ticked off some of the boxes on the form, almost making a hole in the paper with his irritated penmanship.

'What does Matron say? Surely it's her job to check on us and give instructions.'

'That's it, it isn't. They don't want Matrons any more. Think they're old fashioned. It'll be a sad, sad day for the NHS when Matron is gone and is replaced with some over-paid bureaucrat.'

'What do you want me to do, Charge Nurse?' I asked as I drained my cup.

'Make up some dressing packs with the other girls and tidy the cupboards – oh no, wait, let me see what the form says to do in the event it's a quiet night. Oh, I see, bugger all – because the idiot who wrote this has never done a day of real hard work in their petty little lives,' Andrews spat.

By half past ten it was still quiet. Just a few walk-ins with the usual cuts, bruises and burns that needed a quick dressing, but no constant stream of ambulances rushing through our doors with emergency cases like usual. Andrews had calmed down from receiving the new administration forms and shoved them to the bottom of the filing tray to do later – out of sight, out of mind.

'It's all a bit eerie without the drama, isn't it?' said Andrews as he dunked another bourbon into another cup of tea. 'Oh, spoke to soon,' he said, as he popped the whole soggy biscuit into his mouth and we watched a burly middle-aged man with blood dripping down his face stagger into Casualty.

'Oh, that's Alf,' I said, jumping to my feet.

'Who?'

'The landlord from the Adam & Eve,' I told him as I rushed to help Alf to a chair. 'Alf, what's happened to you?'

'One of the Cassidy boys refused to pay his tab. So I told him to pay up or I'd call the Old Bill, and he smashed me in the face with a glass,' he explained.

I looked at his face. It was covered with cuts and bruises, but worst of all above his eye was a deep cut, dripping with blood.

'Oh, Alf. That's a deep cut. You're going to need stitches, I'm afraid,' I told him as I started to clean the wound.

'Just stitch me up and send me on my way, Nurse. I've got a pub full and I need to keep my eye on the till or the takings are always short.'

'I think you'll need to stay in for tonight; we'll need to keep an eye on you,' I coaxed.

'No need for that. Just patch me up and send me on my way,' insisted Alf.

'Hill's right,' said Andrews. 'That's a very nasty cut. I'll call the doctor; just wait and see what he says.'

But Alf shook his head. He was adamant he was going back to the pub. Even after the doctor had sewn the wound up and advised him not return to work he wouldn't listen. It was with a heavy heart I brought him the 'against medical advice' form to sign so he could discharge himself, and with hardly any patients coming in I couldn't help but worry about him once he'd gone.

I didn't have to worry for too long because at eleven o'clock Alf came back in – the wound was still bleeding as he wouldn't stop working to give it a chance to heal. Again, he refused to be admitted and discharged himself, saying he had to get the pub ready for a big do the next day. But when he came back at midnight because he could barely see for all the blood I wasn't taking no for an answer.

'Alf, you're being admitted and don't argue with me,' I told him firmly.

'Yes, Nurse,' he replied like a meek little lamb as I cleaned his wound for the final time. This huge burly man, who could knock seven bells out of a Cassidy brother if needs be, followed me as good as gold to get his pyjamas on and into bed. When I'd sorted Alf out and returned to Casualty, Andrews was once again smirking at me with his arms folded across his chest, grinning from ear to ear.

'Hill, I didn't realise you were such a fierce dictator,' he said. I blushed and got on with sorting out the bandages in the cupboard. 'Well done, Hill. We'll make a harridan of you yet,' Andrews teased.

At six o'clock in the morning we'd still not had one emergency case brought in by ambulance. 'I've never known anything like it,' said Andrews, yawning. 'God, it's hard to stay awake when nothing much is happening. I'll never complain about a frantic night in Casualty again.'

The New Arrival

The reception phone rang. 'I'm not saying I wish harm on anyone, but if this isn't at least an overturned milk van resulting in an air lift I'm going to be very disappointed,' he joked as he picked up the receiver.

I watched Andrews's face as he listened to the caller and then cried out, 'What do you mean, are we open? We're always open. We're a bloody hospital.' He listened open-mouthed and then put the receiver back down. 'Would you Adam and Eve it?' he shouted. 'Some little sod with a plummy voice made a hoax call saying Casualty was closed tonight and all the ambulances have been going to the London or Bart's. Stupid fools didn't even phone here to check. God, I'd like to see the managers' new directive for dealing with this one!'

As I crawled up the staircase to our flat that morning I was glad to be coming off nights and looking forward to some sleep and a day off before going back onto days. I quietly turned the key in the lock and tiptoed into the flat, which was still in shadow as the curtains were drawn and Maddox and Lynch were still snoozing. I pulled back the curtain on my own small room and let out a scream. There was a naked man asleep in my bed. My flatmates tumbled out of their beds, half asleep, and hastily stumbled over to see what had happened. I'd darted to the kitchen and armed myself with a bashed-up saucepan.

'Who the hell is he?' shouted Lynch.

The man rolled over and saw three angry girls staring down at him. I was brandishing the saucepan, Lynch a vase from the coffee table and Maddox a thick rolled-up copy of *The Shrew*. He looked petrified and pulled up the duvet of my bed to cover his hairy chest. I heard the toilet flush and in strolled Wade from the bathroom dressed in a short cream silk slip with green lace trim.

'What's all the screaming about? You scared me half to death!' said Wade.

I looked at Wade and then back at the man in the bed. I squinted in the darkness and then asked, 'Ernie?'

'That's right, Sarah. How you keeping?' he said cheerfully as I dropped my weapon.

'Wade, what is Ernie doing sleeping in my bed?' I shouted.

'Well, the sofa's a bit small for the two of us,' Wade sniggered.

I closed my eyes in disgust. Wade and Ernie in my bed. I stormed off to the bathroom and slammed the door. I heard Lynch say through gritted teeth, 'Get your things and get out, Ernie.'

I heard the front door open and close. Had I overreacted? Was I just being little Miss Prim and Proper? Then there was a knock at the bathroom door.

'Yes,' I said.

The door opened and there were Maddox and Lynch in their nightdresses, both with their arms folded across their chests.

'Wade and that man have gone. You can come out now, Hill,' said Maddox.

'Did I overreact?' I asked meekly.

'No. That was disgusting,' spat Lynch. 'She's got to go.'

'Yes, we want her out by the end of the week,' agreed Maddox.

'And you can tell her tonight,' Lynch told me.

Maddox and I waited while Lynch scanned the shelves of the off-licence, looking for the best bargain. We'd arranged to meet Wade at the Bengal Tiger so the condemned woman could at least have a hearty meal.

'What do you fancy, red or white?' asked Lynch as her fingers picked up a bottle of red.

'You choose,' I said as she took the bottle to the counter.

'Why don't they serve wine in the restaurant?' said Lynch.

'I don't think they have a licence,' I replied.

'They don't want a licence,' snapped Maddox. 'They're Muslim – they don't drink alcohol.'

At the Bengal Tiger, Mr Ahmad was really pleased to see us and gave us a lovely table. I'd decided that I couldn't accept a free meal but nurses often got discounts so I'd ask for that when the time came. Lynch poured the three of us a glass of wine. I kept my eyes on the door waiting for Wade to make her entrance. Yes, I knew she was brash and loud, that she often said and did the wrong things – but I liked her. She made me laugh; I had a good time with her.

'You know why Home Sister chucked her out of the nurses' home,' said Maddox nibbling on one of the huge stack of poppadums Mr Ahmad had given us.

'Why?' I asked, though it wasn't a leap of the imagination to guess why. I'd lived in the room next to her for two years and the walls weren't that thick.

'Caught sneaking a man in,' said Maddox.

'Big deal. They'd have to chuck out half the nurses if they got rid of everyone for that,' said Lynch.

'Yes, but the other girls have got more sense than to come in drunk, singing at the top of their lungs in the middle of the night and dropping their undergarments up the staircase.'

'Where is she supposed to go?' I asked weakly.

'She's been living off us for weeks, Hill. We don't have the room and we can't relax in our own home with all her shenanigans,' Lynch told me. She was right, of course.

We were already on the main course by the time Wade sauntered in. Maddox and Lynch excused themselves to go to the toilets and glared at me in a way that said, tell her and tell her now. Wade flopped down opposite me and, casting a suspicious eye over the delicious dishes on the table, poured herself a large glass of wine.

'I don't think curry is going to catch on,' said Wade, wrinkling her nose. 'Do you think they'd make me egg and chips?'

I ignored her. I was not going to insult Mr Ahmad's generosity by asking for egg and chips.

'Wade, I need to talk to you,' I gulped.

'Yes, pet?' she said, dipping just the tip of her little finger into a dish and placing it cautiously to her lips.

'I'm afraid you'll need to be out of the flat by the end of the week.' Wade just raised one eyebrow. She didn't say a word. 'I'm sorry,' I continued. 'Finding you'd snuck Ernie in was the last straw for the girls, and you were only supposed to be with us temporarily.' She still said nothing, just looked at me with those big painted eyes of hers. 'Obviously, I don't want to see you out on the streets. If you need some money to help you get started somewhere …' My words drifted off. What was I doing?

Wade sucked on her finger, her face still like ice. Then she creased up laughing at me. 'Oh, Hill. You and those nice manners of yours. Anyone else would have chucked me out on my ear a long time ago. Don't fret, pet. I'll be gone by the end of the week. I know you'd let me stay until it was time to draw my pension if it was just down to you.'

'Do you have anywhere to go?'

'I can move in with Ernie.'

'Are you sure? You haven't known him very long. Will it be convenient?'

'Well, it had better be. We're getting married,' she announced.

My mouth dropped open. Wade was marrying Ernie, a Jewish saxophone-playing cab driver, sixteen years younger than her.

When Maddox and Lynch came back from the toilets I could see this was not the scene they'd been expecting – Wade looking jubilant and me with my mouth open like a goldfish. They looked quizzically at me.

'Wade is marrying Ernie,' I said quietly.

They both stared on in blank disbelief too.

'Aren't you going to congratulate me?' she asked.

We all muttered congratulations. Lynch was the first to pull herself together.

'When's the big day?' she asked breezily. Wade was soon going to be someone else's problem – permanently.

'Oh, it won't be for a while yet. He's got to save up for the wedding and he's only in some grotty digs and he wants to find a nice place to start a family.'

'Start a family?' spluttered Maddox in horror before her brain had fully engaged with her tongue.

'Yes, start a family,' snapped Wade. 'I'm in perfect working order, thank you.'

Maddox mumbled an apology.

'Does it matter that you're not … you know?' attempted Lynch.

'What? That I'm older, divorced, a mother and a Catholic?'

'Well, yes,' shrugged Lynch.

'All of the above. But none of that matters when you're in love, does it? And besides, the reason we'll have to wait a while is I'm going to become a Jew.'

'Will they let you?' asked Maddox.

'If Elizabeth Taylor can do it, so can I,' said Wade defiantly.

I couldn't help but laugh. Maddox and Lynch may have got Wade out of the flat, but, as usual with Wade, even when she was down on her luck she still managed to get the upper hand – you couldn't help but admire her for that.

24

I shook my head as I looked at the new student nurses I'd
been sent. Skirts too short, visible holes in their stockings,
watches on the wrong side of their uniforms, hair not properly pinned up, and painted fingernails for crying out loud.
If Sister Raphael saw them they'd be in very hot water. I
don't know what Sister Powell thought she was doing sending them to do an afternoon's practical in the Intensive Care
Unit; they were neither use nor ornament.

'Did you even look in the mirror before you left the
nurses' home this morning?' I reprimanded. 'In your break
you can go and smarten yourself up.'

'Yes, Staff Nurse Hill,' muttered young Winston, tears
welling up in her eyes.

If that makes her cry she won't last till Christmas, I
thought. When she was out of sight I couldn't help but
smile. It wasn't so very long ago it was me that was getting
a ticking off for incorrect uniform. Even on the day I became
a fully registered nurse, back in April, Matron had scolded
me. There were just six of us who completed our nurse
training from my set. There's was no big ceremony, we just

lined up in a row in Matron's office and she gave each of us a frilly nurse's cap. When she came to me she said,

'Congratulations, Nurse Hill. When the Queen gives you a medal you can wear it on whichever side you like. Until then I suggest you remember to pin your watch to the right side of your chest.'

I'd been honoured when Sister Raphael had asked me to come and Staff for her in the hospital's newly opened Intensive Care Unit. The standard of nursing was very high and we had the very latest equipment. The past six months there had been thrilling, but I wanted a change. I went to my small desk and opened the drawer and took out my application. I'd already completed it, and today was the final day to get it in if I wanted to start Obstetrics at the beginning of next year on the Maternity Unit. It was the stepping stone I needed to become a health visitor.

Becoming a health visitor would mean a big change, as Miss Knox had told me over a curry at the Bengal Tiger only last week – I'd be leaving the hospital and then most likely leaving Hackney. I'd never be a sister; I'd never work on the wards again. It would mean saying goodbye to all my friends, my home and the life that meant so much to me. But I would have another year in Hackney to train in Obstetrics, and who knew if I'd even be accepted on the following year's health visitor course. Miss Knox had told me that last year 500 nurses had applied for the forty places – the competition was fierce. If accepted, I'd not only be sitting practical and academic exams, but I'd be studying psychology, sociology, epidemiology, statistical analysis, public health and social policy, and child development as well. Miss Knox told me there were even drama lessons to practise different scenarios we'd encounter in community practice. I'd be up against senior nurses with years more experience than me – hadn't I observed for myself that the health visitors on the district were at least forty, or usually much older. So, say I got onto Obstetrics but was rejected for heath visiting – where would that leave me?

I looked at my nurse's watch. Sister Raphael had given me the afternoon off so I could go to Wade's wedding at the town hall; we'd decided we'd have to go on calling her Wade like an actress, it would be too strange to call her Goldberg. If I left at two o'clock I would have enough time to go home and change for the wedding and pick up Wade.

She'd spent the night at our flat so Ernie wouldn't see her the night before the wedding. Wade had insisted on going out on the town for her last night of freedom. Alf had done a lock-in at the Adam & Eve, and Wade, Lynch, me and even Maddox had stumbled back to the flat at one o'clock in the morning, singing 'I'm Getting Married in the Morning'. We'd unfortunately woken up some of the neighbours. When one old lady had told us to pipe down Wade lifted her skirt and showed her drawers – pointing her behind to the moon.

'Isn't she the blushing bride?' remarked Lynch.

Then at three in the morning we'd been woken by shouting. We'd opened the window to see the flat across the street on fire.

'Oh, God. I think we'll have to evacuate,' shrieked Maddox.

'Do you think we should see if they need any medical help?' I asked.

Wade rushed around trying to save her wedding dress from smelling of smoke by locking it away in the bathroom with the door shut.

'A right mess I'll look tomorrow if I don't get my beauty sleep. At this rate I'll turn up smelling like a kipper as well,' huffed Wade.

'Where's Lynch?' I asked.

'She won't get up,' said Maddox.

'What?' I drew the curtain on Lynch's room. 'Get up, Lynch. There's a fire over the road!'

'When it spreads to here tell me and I'll consider getting up,' said Lynch without opening her eyes and pulling the blankets over her head. 'And keep the noise down, would you.'

Fortunately the fire brigade turned up and got everyone out, and thankfully no one was hurt. The old lady across the street's electric fire had caught alight. As I'd left the flat that morning, Wade was steaming the bathroom, trying to get rid of the slightly barbecued flavour that had stuck to her wedding dress, and looking blurry-eyed, while Lynch looked like a freshly picked daisy.

* * *

Time to do checks on the patients, I thought, as I put my forms away and went to the first bay. Three of the four beds were empty. Lying on crisp white sheets in a bed with a heart monitor beeping at his side, under small high windows, was my bus conductor, Clifford.

'How's my favourite patient this morning?' I asked.

'I'll be as right as rain in no time,' he said weakly. 'Thanks to you and the doctors.'

'That's what we're here for,' I told him cheerfully.

He'd had a heart attack on the bus during the journey to the hospital only last week. When I saw them rush him in I was grateful to be on duty, grateful that the NHS he'd prized so highly and the staff he'd been so kind to over the years had been able to save him.

'I want you to meet my son,' he told me with a wink. 'He's studying to be an engineer. I think the two of you would hit it off,' he laughed, patting my hand.

'I'm not supposed to fraternise with patients or their family members,' I told him with a smile. 'You'll get me into trouble.'

'You got that wedding this afternoon?'

'Yes. Three o'clock at Hackney Town Hall.'

'Well, if you catch the bouquet we'll know it's meant to be. I want to hear all about it tomorrow. You have a good time; you work too hard.'

'I'll see if I can sneak a piece of wedding cake in for you,' I told him as I finished my checks.

'Oh yes. And if it came with a drop of rum that would be even better,' he chuckled.

'Don't push your luck,' I told him as went to check on the other patients before doctors' rounds.

Maddox, Lynch and I lined up on the steps of Hackney Town Hall as we waited for Wade and Ernie to emerge. I wore a black jacket with a large peachy-coloured collar and a matching brimmed hat and skirt my dad had bought me for my sister Bridget's wedding.

'Did you almost laugh the first time you heard the registrar say Edie and Ernie?' asked Lynch.

I grinned and nodded. There weren't too many of us in the wedding party. Despite Wade's recent conversion to Judaism only Ernie's brother, Eric the theatrical agent, turned up from his side. Wade's son couldn't get leave, and was somewhere off the coast of Gibraltar, and I didn't know if she asked any of her family but none of them were there. I recognised a few familiar faces from down the pub but it was a small crowd. A photographer was hanging about, offering to capture people's pictures as they emerged as man and wife. When Ernie and Wade descended the steps he snapped away at Wade's veil fluttering in the wind, her long chestnut curls blowing about her radiant face. She wasn't the least bit embarrassed about wearing white for her second marriage. Ernie was less traditional in a brown suit with an open-necked shirt and sunglasses. Wade turned round and tossed her bouquet over her head towards us girls. It was Lynch who caught it. I was surprised to see Lynch blush, surprised by how pleased she looked.

In true Hackney style Ernie drove his new bride in his cab to the reception in the upstairs room of the Adam & Eve, where we had our Women's Lib meetings. The rest of us were supposed to follow on the bus. As we sauntered along to the bus stop with confetti in our hair it felt like something had changed somehow. Lynch was still grinning at her flowers and surprisingly Maddox wasn't giving us a sermon about how marriage is an outmoded institution purely for the servitude of women.

'Where are they going on honeymoon?' asked Maddox.

'Brighton,' I replied. 'Is Gerald coming to the reception?' We hardly ever saw him. He never came over to the flat.

'He's away at the moment,' Maddox reluctantly volunteered.

'Where is he?' I asked.

'At home,' she told me, but she wouldn't look at us. Even Lynch came out of her reverie, realising something was up with Maddox.

'Is something wrong, Maddox?' I asked.

'Yes and no. You see – I'm moving out.'

'Moving out?' Lynch and I asked in unison.

Maddox nodded and for once looked uncertain about what she was doing.

'To live with Gerald?' cried Lynch, having worked it out.

'Not like that,' said Maddox with a look of horror on her face. 'You see, Gerald's been working very closely with the vicar at St Barnabas. He's decided he wants to take Holy Orders. He wants us to work with the people who really need us.'

'Are you getting married?' I asked her gently.

'I'm going to Rwanda,' she told us breathlessly. 'With Gerald.'

'Are you going to be a missionary?' screeched Lynch with surprise.

'I'm going to go with him and see what happens,' Maddox tried to explain. I'm not sure she knew herself just what she was doing.

'That's a very big step, Maddox,' I said.

'Yes, but sometimes we have to take big steps to find out who we really are,' responded Maddox.

'When are you going?' asked Lynch.

'Next month,' replied Maddox. 'Look, I've got a lot to do and I feel a bit headachy, I might skip the reception and go back to the flat.'

Maddox scurried off and instead of catching the bus Lynch and I decided to walk. It had been a funny day. When we came to the hospital we both stopped and looked at the nurses' home – our old stamping ground.

'Everything's changing, isn't it?' I said to Lynch.

She nodded. There were a group of housemen standing around in a little group. Some were smoking, others sharing sandwiches and crisps on the lawn. One of them was Dr Guy Fleming. He saw us and Lynch hid the bouquet shyly behind her back.

'Hill, I've got to tell you something too,' she said in a whisper. 'Guy's asked me to marry him and I've said yes.'

She looked into my face, worried about seeing the same uncertain reaction we'd both experienced to first Wade's and then Maddox's news. But I was thrilled for her. I hugged her and told her how wonderful it was. Dr Guy's a nice chap and he's lucky to have her, I thought. I saw Dr Guy smiling in the distance and I told her to go and tell him that it's official and there's no going back on it now or he'd have me to answer to.

I crossed the road to the Adam & Eve. Outside the pub was a red post box. I took out my Obstetrics application tucked away in my handbag and held it in my hand. I took a deep breath. This was it – all change.

25

Travelling from our flat to the hospital on winter mornings called for courage at the best of times, but in January 1974, when Heath's government introduced the three-day week once more – so businesses using high levels of electricity could only operate on three consecutive days – I found myself walking to the bus stop without a single street lamp to light the way. It felt like I was a character in a Sherlock Holmes novel making her way through the East London streets. Yet here we were in the mid-seventies. For half the week life was full of colour, we were dancing in discos to Alvin Stardust, and then a switch was flicked and we were reduced to living by candlelight, in a dim, drab world that seemed to be going backwards not forwards. Hope was draining away, the optimism of the sixties straining under the weight of rising prices and reduced wages.

It was just me and Lynch in the flat now – Maddox had left for a life in Africa with Gerald. Wade was finally settled with Ernie in a little house in Clapton Pond and Lynch and Dr Guy had set a date for their wedding in the autumn. It felt like time was being called on our carefree single life. The flat which we'd loved so much was now cold; we were forced to sleep in layers of jumpers and read books by candlelight when the television broadcasts stopped at 10.30 pm. I had to fill a thermos with boiling water before bed to make a tepid cup of tea in the morning. It had been an adventure at first, but as we plodded on into late January the Victorian lifestyle had lost its appeal. It wasn't romantic; it was boring, miserable, freezing and dangerous. Most of our neighbours had been broken into, and even at hospital, where we were supposed to be exempt from the cuts, we were operating by emergency lighting and rubbish was stacking up. The wards were becoming overcrowded with more accidents and illness, and often with people just seeking shelter, warmth and light.

Working in the Maternity Unit to do my Obstetrics training was like starting out all over again. I worked on the Antenatal, Labour and Maternity wards and I had new colleagues, and new ways of doing things. There was a strict hierarchy and I was definitely at the bottom of the pile once more. It was a bit of a shock to go from being a highly thought-of Staff Nurse on Intensive Care to a barely noticed pupil midwife back on student's wages. Both my pride and my bank balance were suffering from the switch to Obstetrics; I just hoped it would stand me in good stead when I made my health visiting application in the spring. I just had to keep my head down and learn as much as I could. Don't make any waves, not even a ripple, I kept telling myself.

Fortunately for me there was one friendly face, as I found myself working with Wade for the first time. I was pleasantly surprised to see how competent she was as a midwife. The mothers loved her down-to-earth humour and directness.

It was strange to sit at the back of the room and observe Wade's antenatal class. I watched each pregnant woman come in. Some were early and took up seats at the front of the class, ready and eager to learn, sitting neatly with their hands folded in their laps on top of a notebook and pen, their handbags tucked under their seats, their coats and scarves folded on the back of their chairs. Others came in laughing and joking in gangs and spread out their belongings on a clutch of chairs, claiming a little patch for themselves. They shared sweets, swapped stories and complained loudly about sore backs and swollen ankles.

Wade strode in, on time, with a doll the size of a newborn baby tucked under her arm, and sat in front of the class. She smiled broadly at the expectant faces in front of her and waited for the chatter to die down. A woman in the front row shot a group of gossiping women at the back a withering glance and shushed them.

'Good afternoon, ladies,' Wade said clearly. 'Now, before we begin, a few little reminders. If you feel the call of nature, just go. The lavatory is back through reception to the left of the main desk. If anyone has any questions don't be a wallflower, do ask. And if it's something you'd rather not mention in front of everyone, then have a little word with me after class.'

A couple of women rushed in late, apologising, and took up seats on the edges of the room. They were smartly dressed in jackets and court shoes, and their hair was fixed in tightly wound buns. Wade smiled and continued.

'Today, we'll be following on from last week's discussion on putting together your layette and bathing a newborn to breast and bottle feeding. I know you might have some more questions on labour and delivery so we can make time for that if you like.'

Wade scanned the room of nodding women and girls – all first-time mums, I was sure they could probably think of very little else as they were only weeks away from giving birth. Wade smiled and continued, 'Then we'll break and have a cup of tea and a chat. And I'll leave plenty of time for your favourite bit of the class – a lie down and some gentle relaxation.'

A woman in a colourful stripy jumper popped up. 'Sorry, I need a wee,' she mouthed to Wade as she waddled out of the room clutching her round belly.

Wade gave a demonstration of breastfeeding using the doll. Once we got past the giggling, embarrassment and the odd colourful comment, Wade was able to gently guide the women through their first feed after giving birth. She then did a demonstration of how to make up a bottle and gave a list of the equipment needed to keep the bottles sterile.

A young girl on the second row put her hand up nervously. 'Nurse, my ma says I should breastfeed because it'll stop me getting pregnant again. Is that true?'

Wade smiled. 'How many brothers and sisters do you have, Nancy?'

'Four brothers and three sisters,' answered Nancy.

'I see. Well, you *can* certainly get pregnant if you are breastfeeding,' replied Wade. 'The only way to avoid pregnancy is through using contraception or to not have sex at all.'

'I'll opt for the second one,' shouted one of the women at the back, and the others jeered.

'How long do you have to make them wait?' asked Nancy's young friend.

'There is no definite length of time. Physically it can take a couple of months for you to recover from giving birth. Some women are ready sooner, and for others it might be that some of you find you aren't physically or emotionally ready to have sex again for some time.'

'What do you mean, emotionally?' asked Nancy.

'Having a baby brings a lot of change,' Wade said softly. 'Good change, most of it,' she smiled encouragingly. 'But you have to judge when you are ready to start relations again.'

'Either way you end up paying for it,' shouted one of the mums at the back. 'Damned if you do and he'll damn you if you don't,' shouted another.

'You can always talk about contraception, and anything about you or your baby after you've given birth, with the health visitor.' I almost did a double take – that could be me in a year's time, I thought excitedly.

'I think it's time for a cup of tea, ladies. If you'd like to join me,' suggested Wade as she made her way to the urn.

Afterwards I helped Wade put out mats and cushions. Once the women were in a comfortable position, some lying on their sides, others sitting cross-legged or resting with their backs against the wall, Wade guided them through relaxation and breathing techniques. I thought they'd make a fuss or joke around but everyone seemed pleased to have a rest and some time to just breathe and listen to Wade's gentle suggestions. When they'd finished Wade said to the now calmer group, 'Lying down is all very well, but as midwives discovered during the bombing in the war, the sooner you are up and about after giving birth the less chance there is of blood clots. I'd go so far as to say that moving about during labour is much more effective and less painful than just lying on your back, but don't quote me to Sister on that.'

'What's bombs got to do with it, Nurse?' said Nancy. 'Did they scare the babies out quicker or something?'

'No. Women had to move about much more to find a safe place. Midwives started to notice that when women were active there were a lot less issues after the birth. Women who are up and about during labour, often seem to have a smoother and faster delivery. Personally, the delivery room is the only place I prefer a bolshie woman, especially when she's been on the gas and air. Do what feels right for you, ladies.'

'My ma don't hold with gas and air. She says she never had no drugs and I shouldn't neither. She says I'll come out a drug addict,' said Nancy again.

'Your mother needs bringing up to date,' remarked Wade. 'Gas and air will not make you or your baby drug addicts. It will make labour more manageable and help you stay in control,' she said firmly.

Wade didn't seem her normally bubbly self after the class. In fact she looked a bit green about the gills. I wondered if everything was all right at home with Ernie. After three months maybe the honeymoon was over? Alarm bells started to ring when Wade told me he was working tonight and would I meet her at the Adam & Eve after work for a quiet drink – I didn't think she knew what one was.

For lunch I'd decided to skip the expense and clamour of the canteen and go for a walk around Victoria Park with a homemade sandwich. With Lynch's upcoming departure I'd been saving like crazy just in case I needed to find a deposit for a new flat. I didn't know where I'd be once I finished Obstetrics at the end of summer. As I crunched through the frosty leaves it was nice to be in the sunlight. It felt like I'd forgotten what it was like to bask in its glow. Hackney had been everything to me but now I found myself drifting off into flights of fancy about the open road, wide open spaces and freedom – not being surrounded by unknown faces on crowded, dirty, unlit streets, worried about being mugged or worse, but being somewhere green and fresh and new instead. I drifted off my usual path and looked at the little terraced houses that lined the streets around the park. They looked so cosy and inviting – proper homes with families in them. I wanted to know when I'd have that; if I would have that.

At the end of one pretty terrace I was surprised to find a car yard. 'Lamptey's Top Quality Used Motors' said the sign over the forecourt in large swirly red letters. Lamptey, Lamptey, I muttered to myself, that named sounded familiar, and then I remembered. The used car salesman with kidney stones in my first year on Male Surgical with Daddy Davis. He'd given me his card and told me to go and see him if ever I wanted a car. The card was long gone – stolen along with the rest of my belongings in my handbag ages ago. I wondered if Mr Lamptey would remember me. I started looking at cars on the lot. A man in a brown-checked suit and bright yellow shirt with a red tie came striding out of the little cabin that was a makeshift office.

'Good afternoon and how can Bertie Lamptey help you today?' he called to me. When he got up close he put his hand to his mouth in surprise and then took my hand, shaking it enthusiastically. 'Nurse Hill, isn't it?' I nodded. 'So, you're ready for that motor now and you've come to see old Bertie. Well, well, well. I'd be happy to do you a very good deal, Nurse, a very good deal indeed.'

'I have been thinking about a car, Mr Lamptey,' I said.

Had I? I didn't think I had but now I was here the idea of it seemed appealing, though how on earth I would tax, insure and run it, let alone buy it, was beyond me.

'But, Mr Lamptey, I haven't taken any driving lessons or my test yet,' I confessed. Unless of course you counted Dad letting me drive his car up and down our old driveway.

'Not a problem. You'll save a fortune by learning to drive in your own car,' extolled Mr Lamptey. 'I know some excellent driving instructors that'll give you a very good discount and have you on the open road in a matter of weeks.'

'I just thought I'd take a look,' I said, now wanting to backtrack on coming here; getting a car wasn't a sensible idea at all.

'I've got the perfect car for you, Nurse. Only had one careful lady owner. Hardly any miles on the clock. Here, let me show you.'

Mr Lamptey directed me to a red Austin A40 that had recently had a fresh lick of paint.

'Why not start the engine and go for a little drive?' he suggested, as I slipped into the car and placed my hands admiringly on the steering wheel.

'I've got to get back to the hospital,' I explained. 'It was very nice of you to show me the car. I will think about it.' I swiftly exited the vehicle.

'I'll keep it back for you, Nurse. Safest, best-priced car I've got at the moment. I don't want to see it going to anyone else,' Mr Lamptey told me firmly.

I waved goodbye and hurried back to the hospital. I couldn't get a car, could I?

While I was waiting for Wade outside the hospital I did something I never did – I telephoned Dad from a payphone.

'How much does he want for the car?' he asked – always direct, my father.

'Sixteen pounds,' I replied in a small voice.

'How much can you spare?' he asked back.

I could hear the TV on in the background and my youngest brother Stephen shouting at my mum about his rugby kit. My parents had moved again and, with only Stephen at home and my father working on a new job in the West Midlands, they'd taken a handsome house in the town centre of Stafford. Dad was designing a custom-made country pile in the sticks on some Earl's estate, and Mum had written to me telling me how much she loved living in town and how she'd had it with country living. She hadn't been able to just pop out to the shops for a pint of milk and a packet of cigarettes since we'd lived in Sevenoaks when I'd been a very small child.

I told Dad I only had four pounds I could spare.

He said to me, 'Don't pay more than fourteen pounds for the car. I'll send you ten,' then there was more shouting. 'Stephen, I don't know where your rugby boots are but if I find them on my dining table again it'll be curtains for you, young man,' I heard my father warn my brother as we said goodbye.

* * *

So much for that quiet drink. Wade had taken one look at the saloon bar lit by candlelight, the jukebox out of action, and before she'd even ordered her usual brandy and Babycham she had one of the junior doctors accompanying her on the piano as she sang 'My Old Man's a Dustman' with all the locals joining in. A group of giggling student nurses started moaning about Wade's out-of-date repertoire.

One shouted out, 'It's bad enough I had to do my shopping in Woollies this evening by gas light. Do you think you could sing something that wasn't one of my great-granny's favourites?'

Never one not to meet a challenge, Wade started up a chorus of the Beatles and before we knew it the whole pub was swaying in candlelight to 'I Am the Walrus', but even that was starting to feel like it was from a time gone by.

Wade flopped down next to me. She was still on her first drink. 'I'm starting to think the Beatles are never getting back together,' she said, teary eyed.

I would normally have thought she was tipsy, but she'd hardly had a drop, unless she'd been sneaking drinks when I wasn't looking.

'What's wrong, Wade?' I asked.

'It's Mrs Goldberg to you,' she snapped.

'All right. What's up, Mrs Goldberg?' I tried again.

Wade took a deep sigh. 'I'm pregnant,' she wailed.

I studied her face. Should I congratulate her? She didn't look exactly thrilled. Instead I plumped for being direct.

'Was it not planned?'

Wade gave me a sour look. 'Of course it wasn't bloody planned. I'll be drawing my pension by the time they finish school,' she cried.

'Is Ernie pleased?' I hesitated to ask.

'He's thrilled. They always are. Means they work. Means they've done their job as a man. Well, I've done my bit already, thank you very much. I had my kid; I raised him, stayed chained to the kitchen sink. I thought this was my time now. Now I'm going to be that poor old fat cow,' she sniffed. 'Bloody Ernie,' she hissed.

'Be fair. It's not all his fault.'

'No. You know who I blame?' I shrugged. 'Ted Heath and Father Christmas.'

'You've got me there, Edie,' I said.

'All these power cuts and Christmas parties. It's got Baby Boom written all over it. Mark my words, come August we'll be rushed off our feet on maternity. Only I won't be there. I'll be one of the poor cows in labour.'

'It'll be lovely having a new baby,' I comforted. 'You'll be a lovely family.'

'Goodbye life. Goodbye freedom. Goodbye job,' Wade toasted as she downed her brandy and Babycham.

'It doesn't have to be that way,' I suggested.

'Yes, it bloody does. Mazel tov,' said Wade. 'I need another drink. And get me a bacon sandwich from somewhere, would you, pet.'

26

I managed to reverse my recently purchased red Austin A40 into the parking space next to the test centre without a single fault. I felt like I'd been holding my breath throughout the entire driving test. I waited for further instructions from the examiner. He wore a grey suit and black-rimmed NHS spectacles, and he had a very thin, greying comb-over. He reached down for the tatty brown leather briefcase at his feet and starting rifling through it. I glanced at my watch. It was already 1.30 pm. I was due back on the maternity unit at two o'clock. Why did I have to be on spilt shifts the week of my driving test? As if working morning, afternoon and evening wasn't bad enough.

The examiner looked over and saw me checking the time. He tutted slightly and then said, 'Please turn off the engine, Miss Hill.' I did as I was told.

He slowly rifled through his briefcase some more and then finally produced a picture of a steam train with smoke coming out of the top.

'Can you tell me what this means?' he asked without looking at me as he scribbled some notes on my test sheet.

'Steam train coming – watch out?' I replied with a gulp and a half smile.

His eyes flashed at me with contempt.

'I suggest you learn your Highway Code, Miss Hill. You've failed your driving test,' he informed me.

Before I could say another word he started packing everything up quickly into his tatty briefcase and exiting my vehicle.

Before he slammed the door shut he said, 'I trust there is someone coming who has a driving licence to drive this car home?'

Wade laughed as she drove me to the hospital.

'I can't believe you didn't learn your Highway Code *and* booked your test on a split shift week,' she teased as we whizzed down the high street.

'I know,' I groaned, now safely in the passenger seat. 'You'll have to test me. Everyone will have to test me. When I'm not on duty I will be learning my manned from unmanned level crossings, I promise.'

Wade looked in the rear-view mirror and gave a little wave to Ernie following behind us in his cab.

'Don't be too hard on yourself, pet,' she sympathised. 'If I'd seen it I wouldn't have known it either. It's just luck as to who you get and what you get on the day.'

'Well, as long as it's the only thing I fail today,' I huffed.

'Oh, yes. You had to get your health visiting application in this morning, didn't you. When's the interview?'

'If I get through the first round, the interviews for training are in June,' I told her. 'But even with a recommendation from Miss Knox I don't want to count my chickens. Hundreds apply every year and they only let a handful in. I'm barely out of nappies compared to most of them.'

'Don't doubt yourself, pet. You're a fine nurse and you'll be an even better health visitor. You can come and practice on me when the bairn comes,' she smiled, pressing a hand to her belly.

At twenty-two weeks Wade had a firm small bump, and she really didn't look her age – she looked marvellous. And as for Ernie, he was walking around like the cat that got the cream. They were a funny pair, but their hearts were in the right place – they were dropping my car safely back to the Balls Pond Road once they'd delivered me to hospital.

Suddenly Wade started signalling madly to Ernie to pull over. 'I'll just nip in here. Baby's desperate for a salt beef bagel,' she told me, pulling up sharply outside a kosher bakery.

'Get a loaf for me,' I called through the window as she disappeared into the shop.

I loved kosher bread; I could have that for supper with butter and a cuppa during my half-hour break at four o'clock. The run-up show to the Eurovision Song Contest would be on. What better way to spend the weekend? Stupid spilt shifts.

* * *

I darted from room to room in Antenatal. I had three women lying in, all waiting to be transferred onto the promised land of Labour Ward. Poor Mrs Mandal had been there since I came on duty at seven o'clock in the morning. Now, at seven o'clock in the evening, she was still there. I checked again to see how far she was dilated; the poor woman was still at seven centimetres, the same as she'd been for the past few hours. She looked hopefully at me as I finished the exam. I could only give her a half smile and shake my head.

'I'm sorry, Mrs Mandal. Baby's still not quite ready to make an appearance yet. Not much longer now. Can I get you something to drink or help you go to the toilet?'

She started to scream, 'I want it out. Get it out. All the other women are in and out – why am I still here?'

'First babies do often take longer,' I soothed. 'You're doing really well. Do you want me to help you walk around a bit to see if we can get things going, or what about a nice bath?'

'A bath,' she said feebly.

'I'll be two ticks. I'll run the bath and then come back and get you.'

I passed Sister Brockman shuffling down the corridor as she came off duty. She cocked her head thoughtfully to one side when she saw my anxious face, and stopped me.

'How's Mrs Mandal getting on, Hill?'

'She's still not progressing, Sister,' I replied. 'I'm just going to run her a bath.'

'Good idea. Why not try getting her to massage the breasts to activate the milk supply. Bit of an old wives' trick but it usually helps move things along,' she told me in a low voice.

When I went back to fetch Mrs Mandal she was on her knees. I helped her up and she leant on my shoulder for support. I held her hand and slowly walked her to the bathroom. I helped her gently get into the bath. When she was lying back in the warm water and had relaxed a little I showed her what to do.

'Right, Mrs Mandal, try placing your fingers at the top of the breast. Now press down slowly, keep the pressure up, that's right, and work your way steadily to the end of the nipple.' She started to do it. 'That's right, keep going. Now try the other side.'

Fifteen minutes later I helped her out of the bath and she had an enormous contraction before I'd even got her dressing gown back on. Before we reached the door she had another contraction and then another.

'Right. Let's get you onto Labour Ward, shall we?' I said.

She looked up at me and nodded furiously. An hour later she safely delivered a little girl.

Mrs Mandal was right about one thing. The other rooms were changing occupants frequently. Many of the mothers were on a fourth or fifth baby and there was just time to catch the newborn after transferring them onto Labour Ward. As I dashed from room to room it was the usual scene in Antenatal: fathers pacing up and down, or Sister having a row with anxious parents because the woman had come in with Braxton Hicks or too early in her labour to be admitted, or the whole family had turned up with toddlers and small children who couldn't be accommodated.

The ward was a sea of constantly changing faces. The whole spectrum of human emotions played out in one small waiting area: hope, happiness, anticipation, fear, anger, jealousy, envy, despair, pride, apathy and contentment.

I was en route to the staff room to take my break when a face I recognised caught my attention – it belonged to Mrs Begum, and she looked most anxious. She was sitting in the waiting area with her arm around a small pregnant Asian woman who was displaying that commonest of emotions when pre-term pregnant women come to Antenatal – fear.

'Hello, Mrs Begum,' I called as I walked over to them.

'Nurse Hill,' she replied with a smile. I was pleased she remembered me. 'Do you work here on the Maternity Unit now?'

'Yes. Can I help?'

'Please. I've brought my friend, Mrs Choudhury, in. She's only thirty-two weeks pregnant but something isn't right. We've been to see the doctor and he says it is just heartburn but she thinks something is wrong. I do too. So I brought her here; I didn't know what else to do.'

'Mrs Choudhury, would you like to come with me into a room and I'll check your blood pressure and then fetch Doctor?'

'She doesn't speak any English, I'm afraid,' Mrs Begum told me.

Once we were in the privacy of a side room I asked what the problem was, with Mrs Begum acting as translator. I took out the cuff and put it round her arm and started to take her blood pressure and listened to Mrs Begum.

'My friend works as a machinist. She has a small sewing machine at home and is paid a few pence per item by one of the big factories. She has to work very long hours to make any money. Her husband works as a kitchen porter at the Bengal Tiger. For the last few days she hasn't been able to work. She is still being sick, Nurse. She gets dizzy and has headaches. She's very worried for her baby. It's her first child.'

'I see,' I replied. This didn't sound good to me. 'Your blood pressure is on the high side, Mrs Choudhury; 160/100. I'm just going to find Sister and get a doctor to come and examine you. Could you do a urine sample for me?'

I waited in the corner of room while the consultant gave Mrs Choudhury a perfunctory examination. Sister Kennedy was at his elbow, giving me daggers with her steely blue eyes as I tested the urine sample. There was a high level of protein in her urine; surely doctor would admit her for observation.

After only a few minutes Dr Plummer said to Sister Kennedy, 'Just another over-anxious mother wasting my time and the NHS's valuable resources.'

Sister nodded in agreement. 'Discharge the patient,' she informed me.

'But her blood pressure, Doctor?' I prompted.

He tutted at me. 'As always pupil midwives can't be relied upon to take blood pressure,' he barked at Sister Kennedy and then stalked off without a by your leave.

Sister Kennedy glared at me. 'What do you think you're doing? If we admitted every mother with a little bit of nausea we'd have half the women in Hackney in residence. Don't presume to tell me or the doctors our jobs.'

'But, Sister …'

'Enough. Get back to the women that actually need your attention,' she told me, and stormed off leaving Mrs Begum opened mouthed at their rudeness.

Mrs Choudhury didn't need anything translating, she knew when she was being blamed for something that wasn't her fault, and became very tearful.

'Best you go home and rest,' I said to her. 'Watch her closely. If anything gets worse bring her back in,' I told Mrs Begum as they left.

She gave me a weak smile and helped her friend walk unsteadily out of the Maternity Unit. Damn them, I thought, as I stamped my foot. That mother knows something is wrong – why won't they listen to her? Soon I had to put thoughts of Mrs Choudhury out of my head for the final hour of my shift, but as I waited for the bus on Homerton High Street to take me home I wondered if I could talk to Sister Brockman about it.

★ ★ ★

The next day, even though it was a Saturday afternoon, Sister Brockman couldn't resist giving a little tutorial during a rare quiet hour on the Antenatal Ward. I'd asked her about possible pre-term conditions in pregnant women with high blood pressure. She was a small woman, with a rounded back and shuffling walk. Despite being well into her sixties, her hair was still black except for white wisps that lined her centre parting. When it came to newborn babies she never grew tired of having a quick cuddle, but if you crossed her she soon bared her teeth and gave you a dressing down. So, to no surprise, her pupils called her The Badger.

Sister Brockman was following on from the Obstetricians lessons the previous week on the complications during premature labour. Just thinking about them made me give a little shiver as I thought of all those hopeful mothers who just wanted to come out of hospital with a healthy baby in their arms. I was still worried about Mrs Choudhury.

Unfortunately, The Badger's memory wasn't what it was, and as teatime drew near she finished her lecture with her customary, 'I'll pick up threads later, dear,' which she never did.

As she made her way to the sisters' sitting room she said majestically, 'I don't know why anyone would go private nowadays – money down the drain. The NHS is the best in the world,' and off she sauntered for a cup of Earl Grey and a custard cream.

I strolled into the staff room to take my half-hour supper break. A little huddle of midwives was gathered round a small portable black-and-white set watching the Eurovision Song Contest.

'There, there she is,' cried one of the midwives. 'That's my sister. She lives in Brighton and got tickets to see it.'

'Which one is she?' asked another midwife.

'There. Three rows back behind Sandie Shaw.'

I strolled over and asked, 'Who's representing us?'

'Olivia Newton-John,' answered the first midwife.

'Has she been on yet?' I ventured.

'Yes,' replied the second midwife a bit sourly.

'Any good?' I asked. They both turned and looked at me disdainfully. I retreated back to make my supper.

'Sweden's on next,' the second midwife announced.

My back was turned to the television as I rooted around in the cupboard getting a plate and a cup. I heard the announcer proclaim that Sweden was full of blonde Vikings. Then I heard him say, 'If all the judges were men – which they're not – this group would get a lot of votes and you'll see why in a minute.' I sighed and thought fondly of Maddox and what she'd make of the commentator's comments. Then a group of four singers were shown crouching down behind the large leaves of a big pot plant and peeking up at the camera. 'There's Frida, Anna and Benny. Or rather Anni-Frid, Björn, Benny and Anna – ABBA,' said the commentator smugly. A conductor dressed as Napoleon waved to the audience to a big cheer and two Swedish girls bounced onto the stage and started to sing. One had curly hair and wore a long skirt. The other girl had the better outfit; she had long blonde hair and was dressed in a satin blouse and trousers with huge sparkly knee-length platform boots.

'Gosh, she's a looker,' said the first midwife, pointing at the blonde girl, as ABBA started singing 'Waterloo'.

All the staff in the room were nodding and beating time along with the song. A little group of Irish midwives started to jive along to it.

'You're so old fashioned with your jiving,' sniggered the second midwife.

The announcer remarked at the end of the song, 'Sweden have never won it. But it's gone down well in the Dome here in Brighton.'

'Oooh, there's my sister again,' cheered the first midwife as the camera panned round the audience.

When I'd finished my break I was shocked to find Mrs Begum sitting in the waiting room. She looked fraught as she clung tightly to the sleeping child on her chest. Her cheeks were tear stained and her eyes red and sunken. When she saw me she started to tell me very fast that Mrs Choudhury had woken up this morning to find her legs and feet were very swollen. Her friend was getting pains in her abdomen, and she felt very sick and dizzy and could barely walk. Then this evening her waters had broken and the two women had been alone and so she'd called an ambulance. They rushed her in and took her into theatre to deliver the baby. But she'd heard nothing since and then she thought she'd come and find me to see if I could find out what had happened. She was worried for her friend. How would she understand anyone? How would they understand her?

I immediately sought out The Badger, who gave me permission to go to Labour Ward with Mrs Begum. I found Mrs Choudhury on Maternity. Thankfully her baby had been delivered safely. She'd had a tiny little boy, only 2 lb 11 oz, but he was in no danger and being cared for in an incubator in the special unit for premature babies. But Mrs Choudhury looked terrible. Mrs Begum asked her how she was but the poor woman could barely respond.

'She's not making sense,' Mrs Begum told me. 'She keeps asking, "Did my baby live? Did my baby live?" I don't think she knows what's happened.'

Mrs Begum tried to reassure her friend that her baby was fine but I could tell Mrs Choudhury didn't understand her. She was rambling, surely anyone could see that, you didn't have to speak Bengali.

I took a cuff and started to take her blood pressure but it was so high I could barely get a reading; it was somewhere over 200.

Panic rising in me, I dashed off and begged Sister Kennedy and Dr Plummer to come and see her, but they told me to stop being melodramatic. The baby had been delivered safely, all was well. The mother was just being uncooperative and attention seeking.

I wheeled Mrs Choudhury into a side room and was considering my options. What could I do? Fetch another doctor? Get a second opinion? But before I had the chance to choose a course of action Mrs Choudhury started having a fit. I didn't know what was happening. Was the woman epileptic? I called the crash team and my old friend Sister Raphael from Intensive Care came running with her team to bring Mrs Choudhury round. The seizure went on for a few more minutes, and they felt like the longest of my life.

Thankfully, Mrs Choudhury's fit stopped and she became stable, barely conscious but stable. Sister Raphael said she needed to be transferred to Intensive Care immediately and monitored closely. I felt wrung out. Even during my time as a Staff Nurse I'd never seen anything like it.

'Sister, what was that?' I asked Sister Raphael as they started to wheel Mrs Choudhury out of the maternity ward.

'Toxaemia, Hill. We're lucky she survived,' she said. Then turning to a stunned Sister Kennedy and Dr Plummer she said sharply, 'Very lucky indeed. This warrants a full investigation and at the very least an apology. I'm sad to say we almost completely failed this woman.'

I'd never been so glad I'd made waves. I knew I'd blotted my copy book with Sister Kennedy and Dr Plummer but I didn't care. The whole medical profession had let Mrs Choudhury down, from the GP to the hospital consultant. I promised myself I would never dismiss a mother, never judge by appearances. Mrs Choudhury knew something was wrong but she was pushed aside – just another hysterical woman, like her illness was somehow her responsibility. When it came to women's health we had so far to go. I knew then that I wanted to spend my life helping mothers and their babies right when life begins. Nothing mattered more to me.

27

A flicker of excitement ran through me when I saw the principal of Health Visitor Training, Miss Emmanuel, walk onto the small stage in Maidstone Polytechnic. She was legendary – a diminutive, wiry woman in her sixties with grey, neatly packed curls and a snub nose, who had dedicated her life to community practice. I sat in the middle of the second row – I didn't want to miss a thing. I'd been looking forward to this day; I was ready to take the next step and I hoped that it was a day that would change the course of my life.

I looked from side to side and behind me at the rows of other nurses filling the compact red-brick hall. One or two I'd noticed at Victoria Station and a few more on the bus here. Five rows of eight women were set out in neat lines in front of the stage where Miss Emmanuel stood waiting for hush. Behind her five other senior nurses were seated – they would make up the day's interview panel. I scanned the ranks once more, sizing up the competition; I must have been the youngest woman in the room by at least fifteen if not twenty years. I'd opted for the trusty suit I'd worn for Bridget's and Wade's weddings, though this time without the hat. I slid my peach pencil skirt over my knees after noticing the hemlines around me were considerably longer, and undid the buttons on my jacket in an attempt to cool down. I didn't want my throat to become dry in this stuffy room and be the victim of the Hill tickle. A swift exit from the room in a coughing fit in front of Miss Emmanuel would not do. I licked my lips to moisten my mouth as I waited for our principal to start.

Silence fell. Miss Emmanuel smiled at the nurses below her, showing all her teeth. I could even see the fillings at the back.

'Welcome. Congratulations, ladies, on reaching the interview process. This year the standard has been very high. We received over 400 applications for September's intake, and I'm pleased to say you are among the 200 remaining nurses from all over the country we will be interviewing for the 47 places for Health Visitor Training. The few of you who pass today's interview process can look forward to a rigorous and fulfilling year of training.

'We expect our students to reach the highest academic standards alongside exemplary fieldwork practice. You can expect tough essays and challenging case studies before sitting your final exams. Alongside our assessment of your medical knowledge you will be sitting five three-hour exams to assess your knowledge of psychology, sociology, epidemiology, public health and social policy, as well as your grasp of the practice of health visiting. After twenty hours of examinations, your essays will be marked and added to the scores of your oral exams and individual research projects. So, to summarise, ladies, there will be lots to sink your teeth into.

'Training will begin in the classroom with fieldwork one day a week until Christmas, then two days a week, followed by mid-term exams. Only those who pass through these stages will graduate to a three-month practical placement with a full-time health visitor on a challenging caseload in the community. You will need to be self-sufficient, determined and possess a driving licence. Don't expect much of a social life as weekends will be taken up with study and preparation for seminars. Anyone who is not prepared to dedicate the whole of next year to study and hard work should opt out today and not take up a valuable place on my course,' said Miss Emmanuel, casting a beady eye over the assembled nurses, baring all her teeth, detecting the slightest flinch or rolling of the eyes. I thought she was laying it on a bit thick. Miss Emmanuel made Matron look blithe by comparison.

'You will find,' continued Miss Emmanuel, 'that health visiting is very different to nursing. Nursing is the treatment of the sick. Health visiting is the prevention of ill health. It is more cerebral. You may think you are educated nurses. Well, let me tell you, you are not very educated, you are not well read. You are ignorant. The sooner you accept that, the better. And the more likely you are to succeed in broadening your ideas and understanding of the world.'

Blimey, I thought. Who does she think she is? Calling me ignorant and ill-educated. How right she was.

'It was made crystal clear on the application form, but just in case it slipped anyone's notice, let me repeat; we do not accept women with children under five years of age.' I looked around the room – unlikely, I would have thought, unless of course she was addressing me. I felt her eyes piercing into me. 'We need women who are good under pressure. Who are mature, confident, self-sufficient women, who know how to act and do not hesitate to do so. You will have been used to going to Sister or Matron for guidance. There are no sisters or matrons in the community. You must decide how to act and understand the consequences.'

She made health visiting sound dire. Thankfully, I'd been out with Miss Knox and experienced it for myself, otherwise I might have left early and gone home. I certainly noticed there were fewer candidates at the end of the day than the beginning – perhaps this outcome had always been Miss Emmanuel's intention. I wasn't scared, I was sure her bark was worse than her bite. In the interviews I relished the opportunity to talk about why I wanted to be a health visitor. I wanted it so badly – they just had to accept me.

28

The flat was covered in half-packed boxes. Lynch was sitting in the middle of a cardboard fort, a half-empty glass of red wine in front of her, wearing jeans and one of Dr Guy's stripy shirts. Her hair was in rollers and she had a green face pack on. She was humming along with the radio, The Three Degrees singing 'When Will I See You Again' echoing in the half-empty room. She had a large piece of paper spread out on the floor in front her and was moving little card place names about on it like a general organising battle plans. As I closed the door behind me, she didn't look up; she was frowning at the chart and biting her lower lip in contemplation.

'Hill, do you mind if I put you next to next to Guy's cousin George? Only he went to Harrow and you're the only posh friend I have.'

'No, I don't mind,' I said faintly.

I hovered in the doorway, unsure where to go. There wasn't a place to sit; everything had a box on it and most of our things had already been packed away. I looked at the curtain drawn back on Maddox's former room, revealing only a bare mattress on a rickety bed frame and empty shelves. Soon the whole flat would be like that, as if we'd never even been here.

'What's wrong? Don't be mad I haven't finished the packing. We don't have to be out till Tuesday morning. I'll have it all done by then, I promise,' pleaded Lynch. 'Only I can't face Guy's mother at the end of the week if I don't know where I'm sitting his Great Aunty Edith, I just can't.'

I couldn't reply. I just started to sob huge great tears that wouldn't stop. And the music – I wanted it to stop, I wanted it to all stop. Lynch sprang up and ran to me, wrapping her arms around my shuddering shoulders.

'Can you turn that off, please?' I asked in a small voice.

Lynch immediately silenced the radio.

'What's the matter, Sarah?' she asked softly.

'Oh, Fiona. We lost a mother tonight. We couldn't save her. I just stood there and watched Dr Chakravarti tell the husband she'd died. He looked utterly lost, utterly, utterly lost,' I cried. 'And the baby. The poor baby. And they've got a two-year-old girl as well. That's two little girls without a mother. It's just not right.'

'Did the baby survive?'

'Yes, she did, thank God. The baby was never in any danger; that's why it was such a shock. I've never lost a mother before, never. She just started hyperventilating and then we lost her; they think it was a pulmonary embolism. She didn't even get to hold her baby.'

'These things happen. It's very sad, but it's part of life. There's no way you could have known there was a blood clot on the lung, if that's what happened.'

'I can't be a midwife.'

'Well, you don't have to be. You've got on to that health visiting course; you start in two weeks.'

'I don't deserve it. I don't deserve it. What sort of nurse am I? Why couldn't we save her? Why couldn't we?'

Lynch pressed me tightly to her. 'I once told you not to take it all so personally, do you remember?' I nodded, sniffing as the first wave of tears subsided. 'I was wrong about you, Sarah Hill. It's because you care that you're a great nurse. Hang onto that, Sarah.'

I hugged her. 'I held it together all the way to the flat,' I told her. 'All the way through packing up the mother's things. Taking off her short multi-coloured nightie, her wedding band, and listing it all on the envelope and giving it to the husband before they took her down to the morgue. He just looked at me when I handed it to him, not knowing what to do. I can still see her lying there in the bed, in her nightie, her beautiful black hair spread out on the pillow as he said goodbye to her. I'll never forget her till the day I die. Never,' I wept.

29

It's funny to finish somewhere on a Monday, I thought, as I waved goodbye to Clifford and hopped off the bus onto Homerton High Street for the last time in five years. I took a long look at the hospital before I walked round to the Maternity Unit. My last morning as a Hackney nurse. I couldn't quite believe it, it didn't feel real. How could I be leaving Hackney?

At least my shift finished at six o'clock, so I could do the last bit of packing. Lynch was supposed to be moving out all her things with Dr Guy this morning, if she finished that seating chart in time. And I didn't fancy hanging around tomorrow morning waiting for our landlord Mr Baldini to arrive for a final inspection. No, thank you. I'd be up nice and early to drive to Stafford to stay with my parents for a fortnight before my Health Visitor Training course started in September. And I'd be getting there under my own steam now I'd passed my driving test, I thought with a little thrill of excitement.

I told myself firmly there was no point dwelling on yesterday. I couldn't change it, I couldn't give those children their mother back and I couldn't allow it to stop me doing my job. But I knew it would stay with me like a small scar; the sort you forget about for a while, as life goes on, but then you see it, remember it, and the pain is a fresh as the day you hurt yourself. Don't dwell on it, Sarah, don't dwell on it, I'd told myself earlier as I'd got ready. This isn't your sorrow, it belongs to the husband, the daughters, and you serve no purpose by making it your own. Lynch was right, I knew she was right. Today had to be a fresh day.

It was buzzing on the Maternity Unit. Every midwife seemed to be rushing from room to room. There was an enormous gaggle of fathers, family and friends pacing round the waiting room, and the phone was ringing constantly. Behind the reception desk on the phone was Dr Chakravarti. She waved when she saw me and smiled. Maternity had been a better place in the last few weeks since Dr Chakravarti made the move from Gynaecology to Obstetrics. She was a breath of fresh air and when she was the senior doctor on duty she insisted we worked as a team. She knew every mother in her care, their names, their situations, their preferences. If a woman was brought in pre-term with complications or was having a long labour she would often telephone from home when she was off duty to see how they were progressing. I'd never seen another doctor do this. She treated the midwives like colleagues, and they loved her for it. When she led the team you could see that everyone was nicer to the patients, more confident and competent. But she was in the minority in every sense.

'Busy day today, Nurse Hill,' she told me as she finished her telephone call. 'Every mother from thirty-eight weeks onwards in Hackney seems to have gone into labour today.'

The Badger rushed over. 'Hill, I know it's your last day but there'll be no taking it easy. Labour Ward is frantic. We've barely got enough hands to deliver the babies. I need you to float across all the rooms and use your common sense to manage the women in early labour as best you can.'

I did as I was told and ran from room to room, doing my best to calm things down as we got overcrowded. It wasn't an easy task sending women home who had come in too early to be admitted or getting the women who'd left it a bit too late and were about to deliver on the waiting room floor quickly through to Labour Ward.

After seven straight hours on duty I needed a break, but there just weren't enough of us. As soon as we sent one woman down to Labour Ward and cleaned up the room it was immediately occupied again by somebody else. The Badger popped her head round the door.

'Hill, could you check on a Miss Casebow in room one, please. She's giving the midwives a rather hard time. They might need a few minutes' break.'

I nodded and before I'd even entered room one I heard Miss Casebow shouting at the older midwife attending her.

'How long is this going to take?' she screamed. 'And don't give me no politician's answer.'

'You are still in the early stages of labour. If you could calm down. You'll wear yourself out,' suggested the midwife.

'Don't you tell me what to do. I want you to get this baby out now,' screamed Miss Casebow.

'I can't do that, I'm afraid, dear,' said the midwife. 'Best let nature take its course.'

'Don't talk to me about nature, I'm from Hackney,' she huffed. 'Take me to the toilet, then. I need to go.'

'The toilet's just at the end of the corridor, dear.'

'I can't walk. Get me a wheelchair.'

'It's not too far. I'll help you.'

'I said get me a wheelchair.'

I saw the midwife scurry out to fetch the wheelchair. I was just about to knock and introduce myself when I saw Miss Casebow's mother looking at the gas and air machine. She then took a huge gulp of it.

'It's good, this is, Jenny. You should try it,' said the mother.

I was just wondering what to do when I saw Wade waddling down the corridor with a confused-looking Ernie following behind, carrying two suitcases and a couple of shoulder bags.

'Edie, you all right?' I asked.

'Oh, Hill. I'm getting contractions but Sister Kennedy insists it's just Braxton Hicks.'

'Hello, Sarah,' puffed Ernie under the weight of his wife's luggage.

'Blimey, Wade. What have you got in there? You'll give Ernie a hernia.'

'I'm not having hospital sheets or pillows. And I'm not letting anyone see me in a mess. I've got plenty of clean clothes, my own soaps, make-up, shampoo, conditioner, hair spray, plenty of knickers, some snacks, bottle of gin should things take a turn for the worse.'

'Wade!'

'I'm only joking about the gin, pet. Keep your knickers on.'

'Anything for the baby?' I asked.

'Oh yes. His nibs' mother hasn't stopped knitting since the day we told her. I said to her she needn't bother for a summer baby. I've been down Mothercare already. Anyway, I need a salt beef sandwich. Ernie, you can put that lot back in the cab and drive me to the bakery. I'll be down in five minutes.'

'Righto, Edie,' said Ernie cheerfully as he tried to wave goodbye under the weight of Wade's oversized shoulder bag.

'He's getting on my nerves,' hissed Wade once her husband was out of sight.

'He's doing his best, Edie.'

'I know, I know. I'm a miserable cow. Gosh, it's busier in here than Piccadilly Circus, isn't it.'

'It does seem to have gone a bit mad, yes.'

'What did I tell you? Ted Heath and those power cuts have a lot to answer for. Baby Boom.'

'I better get back to it.'

'You do that, pet. Last day, isn't it?'

I nodded and looked at my nurse's watch, 'Only an hour to go.'

Wade wrapped her arms around me.

'Sarah Hill, it was a good day when you came into my life, turning up in Hackney in your chauffeur-driven car with your boarding school trunk. Don't go changing.'

And she kissed me. Then she cried, 'Braxton Hicks my foot!' as her waters broke in the middle of the antenatal ward.

When my shift finished at six o'clock Wade had been admitted to Antenatal Ward. I was supposed to be packing up the last of my things back at the flat but Wade had begged me to stay with her. Ernie couldn't take the waiting and was circling around the hospital in his cab. The Badger was seeing to Wade personally, no junior midwives or pupils for her, and Dr Chakravarti checked in every hour to see how she was progressing.

Wade was resplendent on the hospital bed, eating from a box of chocolates and flicking through a magazine between contractions.

'I thought you recommended being up and about during early labour?'

'I'm relaxing while I still can,' Wade told me.

The Badger came in and began palpating Wade's abdomen while Wade continued to stuff Dairy Milk down her throat. Sister Brockman sucked her cheeks in and got out the foetal stethoscope shaped like a cornet and listened carefully.

'It's a footling,' she declared.

'I know that. I am a bloody midwife,' huffed Wade.

'Hill, get Dr Chakravarti and see if she can turn the baby,' instructed Sister.

I returned moments later with the ever-calm Dr Chakravarti and took up my place again at the head of the bed with Wade. She didn't offer me one of her chocolates, lying back being waited on like the Queen of Sheba.

'Edie, would you like me to see if I can turn the baby for you?'

'If you would please, doctor,' replied Wade sweetly.

Wade lay back and behaved herself for once as Dr Chakravarti started to palpate on her abdomen.

'You are a few weeks early, so there is a little bit of room in there to try and get your baby to go head down. Sister, please give Edie something to help her relax.'

Dr Chakravarti placed one hand on the baby's head and one on the bottom, getting a firm grip.

'Now, Edie, nice long deep slow breaths for me, and try and relax your body as much as you can. Yes, that's it, good, good,' encouraged doctor as her hands rocked in small motions from side to side as she tried to move the baby round to the right way up.

'Nearly there. You've got a nice cooperative baby here. And there we go,' said Dr Chakravarti smoothly.

'Doctor, I could kiss you,' said Wade.

Dr Chakravarti beamed. 'I'll be back to check on you in an hour but call me if you need me in the meantime.

Hopefully it won't be too long before you can be transferred to Labour Ward. I'm looking forward to meeting your baby, Edie.'

It was nearly midnight. We'd been on Labour Ward for hours. Poor Wade was exhausted. She held my hand tightly and screamed.

'I can't do this any more, I'm too old.'

'Yes you can, Edie. Come on, you're nearly there.'

I looked down anxiously at The Badger at the foot the bed. Wade took another big hit of gas and air. She was so out of it, with only moments of consciousness before the contractions took hold of her again.

'That's it,' encouraged Sister.

Edie lay back exhausted with only a minute to rest before her next contraction.

'You're doing so well, Edie,' I told my friend.

'Edie, we're almost there. When you get the next contraction I want you to push down into your bottom,' said The Badger calmly.

We waited for the next contraction. Edie pushed, almost breaking the fingers on my hand.

'That's it, push, push, push, push,' said The Badger. 'I can see the top of the head peeking through. Nearly there. Give me a really big push with the next contraction.'

Edie was panting with her eyes closed.

'Don't pant, Edie, just push for me. That's it, I can feel the baby's head.'

My eyes met Sister's. Something was wrong.

'The cord is wrapped around the baby's neck,' said Sister in a low voice.

I don't think Wade heard her; she was riding the waves of the contractions and gas and air.

'Hill, I need you to quietly fetch Dr Chakravarti. Don't alarm the mother.'

I quickly returned with the doctor. Edie opened her eyes and saw us all standing at the end of the bed.

'What's wrong?' shouted Edie in a moment of lucidity.

'Edie, I need to get this baby out quickly,' said Dr Chakravarti. 'You've done a marvellous job and we are almost there. There's not quite enough give in the cord as the head came out and it's become wrapped around the baby's neck. Now, I want to get the baby out as quickly as possible. Is it okay if I give a helping hand just to move things along faster and unwrap the cord now?'

Edie had tears in her eyes but she nodded.

Dr Chakravarti reached in. We all held our breath.

'That's it. I've managed to pull the cord over the baby's head. Now I think we are all ready to meet your baby, Edie. When the next contraction comes give me the biggest push you can.'

I could see Edie gritting her teeth and pushing down as hard as she could.

'Push, Edie, push. I'm just guiding the baby out. You are doing beautifully.'

The baby slithered out and Dr Chakravarti quickly handed him to Wade.

'You have a beautiful baby boy,' congratulated the doctor.

Wade was crying as she held her son in her arms for the first time.

'You're the best surprise I've ever had,' she told him as she kissed her newborn son on the top of his purple-coloured head.

I was crying and even Sister and Dr Chakravarti were teary. It was different when it was someone you knew, someone you cared about. Such a beautiful moment.

'You clever, clever girl,' I said to Wade.

She looked up into my face. I'd never seen her look so happy.

'Can you get Ernie, please, Sarah?'

I dashed off and found Ernie. He was sitting alone with his head in his hands in the waiting room.

When he saw me he looked up full of anguish.

'I ran out of petrol,' he said.

'Never mind. Would you like to meet your son, Mr Goldberg?' I asked with a huge smile.

He leapt into the air and I took him through to Wade. As I watched their new family come together for the first time I decided to just gently slip away and let them have those precious few moments together before all Ernie's relatives turned up. It was a good last day as a Hackney nurse.

30

I loaded my old school trunk into the boot of my Austin A40. A few cardboard boxes were stacked on the back seat and I was all packed and ready to go. I'd only had just enough money to fill up the tank to drive me to my parents' place. I posted the keys through the letterbox to the flat and took one last look at the Balls Pond Road. I couldn't believe that I was leaving the East End. I'd loved my five years here; it had welcomed me, changed me and been a home where I felt loved and accepted for who I really was. And now it was over.

I got in my car and turned on the ignition. It didn't make sense to drive past the hospital, it was completely the wrong direction – but I couldn't help it. I turned on the radio.

'Still at Number One, The Three Degrees with "When Will I See You Again",' announced the DJ. I laughed to myself – it was that song again.

As I drove down Homerton High Street I waved goodbye to the hospital, the nurses' home, the Adam & Eve and St Barnabas. I stopped at the traffic lights. A group of young student nurses were laughing as they crossed over the road in front of me.

I thought back to that shy seventeen-year-old who'd arrived in a sulk because her mother had come with her. Who was so eager to make friends and do the right thing. I thought of all my wonderful friends and hoped we'd keep in touch. As I left Hackney I was happy. Happy I'd been there and met so many people who'd changed the way I saw the world for ever. I'd been there at a time when Britain was changing, mainly for the better. I'd become a nurse, a good one, and I couldn't wait to start the next chapter in my life. Imagine all the people I'd meet and things I would learn visiting their homes. Soon I'd be the new girl yet again. It was going to be such fun – my next big adventure. I was going to be a health visitor.

Acknowledgements

Thank you to our literary agent Piers Blofeld, who first suggested writing this story, before it had even occurred to us, and to Paul Magrs for his advice and encouragement. To Charlotte Cole for her speedy copy-editing and practical advice, and to Carole Tonkinson and Anna Valentine at HarperCollins for their alacrity. To Hannah MacDonald for seeing the potential, and Elen Jones for her enthusiasm. To Katie Ormerod at St Bartholomew's Hospital Archives for the illuminating Hackney Hospital records. To John Scanlon, Hotel Manager at the Dorchester, for going out of his way to get us a 1970s menu from the hotel. To Peggy Johnson, Carmel Glennie (née Ryan) and Dr Hugh Glennie for being part of it and for their continued friendship. To William, Jane, Bridget and Stephen Hill and Eric and Margaret Hill for being exemplary parents. And most of all thank you to Takbir Uddin and Ava.

Sarah Beeson (née Hill) and Amy Beeson

Enjoyed *The New Arrival*?
Try *The Midwife's Here!* and *Bundles of Joy*
by Linda Fairley

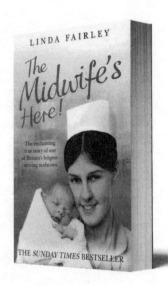
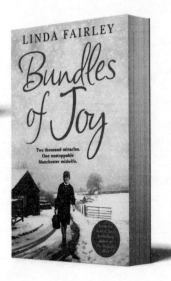

The enchanting true story of one of
Britain's longest-serving midwives

hospital corners I vowed to buy some cotton bed linen as soon as I could. I closed the thin curtain that separated my own tiny cell from the main living space. It was a good feeling – our own place, our own rules. The curtains were still drawn across Maddox's and Lynch's bedrooms as they were both at Nurses' School and only had to attend classes from nine till five. I returned my drained cup to the kitchenette and washed it up. Our modest kitchen was on its last legs and was just about standing. It was propped up against a big window that looked down onto the busy street below. It consisted of no more than a sink, two cupboards, a grill and a two-ring gas hob. Seascapes of Viareggio, with cracked glass or missing frames, were dotted about on the walls. The floors were covered with yellowing grey lino; I'd heard the mice scurrying across it during the night. The furniture was from the 1930s, fading ruby red and emerald green cushions sat on our sunken sofa, we had two armchairs, one with a hole in the seat that I'd covered with an embroidered throw I'd picked up in a junk shop, and the other had a leg that was nibbled by mice or woodworm so it was shorter than the other three and wobbled despite our efforts to prop it up with a bit of cork. Lynch joked we had booby-trapped furniture to get rid of any bad dates. There'd been quite a few of those recently.

I waited at the bus stop. Being December, it still wasn't really light even now at 7.30 am and I felt uneasy as I looked up at the rows the rows of unknown rooms towering above me on both sides of the long grey street. At the nurses' home

I'd met the occupants of most of the rooms, and anyway they were just other girls. Here in this unfamiliar part of town they could be anyone – the wrong side of town, Wade had warned, when I'd told her we were moving out; I think she was a little hurt not to be invited to come with us. I gave a little shiver as I thought of our landlord, Mr Baldini, and his greased black moustache and hair, his shiny grey suit and over-familiar patter, as he'd attempted to discover if we were attached when he'd turned up to hand over the keys the previous afternoon. I'd lied and said I had a boyfriend, but it was Lynch he was really after. I saw him admire her small, neat figure and lively eyes.

'Where are you from, Bella?' he'd asked her.

'Ireland. Are you Italian?' asked Lynch.

'Yes, I came here as a prisoner of war. I like it so much I make my home here.'

'Oh, were the Germans cruel to you?' said Lynch sympathetically.

He smiled at her. Maddox and I rolled our eyes and ushered Mr Baldini out of the flat.

'The Italians were on the side of the Germans,' snapped Maddox once our landlord was out of earshot. 'He was *our* prisoner.'

I was glad when the red bus rolled up and I jumped on the back. The bus conductor gave me a huge friendly grin that made me feel much more at ease.

'And where you off to, darling?' he asked cheerfully.

to; on no account are any of my nurses to share their Christian names with patients or their visitors. The boundaries between nurses and doctors must be maintained too. You are not to address the consultants directly; if there is any discussion needed about a patient you will go through me. Specifically, Mr Duncan will be visiting a child with Perthes disease to monitor his progress ahead of a visit from the mobile X-ray unit in the next few days. This child's mother seems determined to disrupt the running of my ward with a lot of soft notions about children – she is not to be indulged in such mollycoddling.'

'Yes, Sister,' I replied instinctively to She-Who-Must-Be-Obeyed. While she's around at least, I thought.

'It should be a simple enough task for a girl with eight O-levels. You may go, Nurse Hill.'

I was dismissed and eagerly went to find Appleton. I was shocked to find her attending to two toddlers I knew well in steam tents.

'Oh, no. Not Georgie and Bobbie in again?' I asked.

'Afraid so,' replied Appleton. 'Their poor mothers; I think things are worse than ever. They are never going to get over their bronchitis living in that house, and each time they get worse and worse. Where are you off to?'

'TPRs on the little boy with Perthes in bay one.'

'Oh, little Paul Murphy, he's lovely.'

'Anything else I should know about?' I asked.

'Well, there is the mystery of Sister Skinflint's missing egg sandwich,' said Appleton with a wink.

'Hackney Hospital, please,' I said getting out my little purse.

'Put your money away, Nurse,' he said. 'I like to do my little bit to say thank you to the NHS.'

I was grateful and happy to chat as the bus bumped along. He told me proudly about his wife, three daughters, son and mother back home in Jamaica. It made me think about my own parents – I hadn't told them I wouldn't be back for Christmas yet. I hadn't even told them Alex and I had broken up. It made me feel like such a fool after we'd just been home to introduce him to everyone.

I ran up the main hospital staircase eager to start my new stint on Infants Ward. It was funny to think back to that veritable schoolgirl who'd first walked through those doors – playing at being a nurse in her brand-new uniform over two years ago. By now the number of classmates in my set had more than halved, and at twenty I'd reached a maturity on duty that was beyond my years of experience, though off duty my understanding of the world still had a long way to go. I was so happy at the prospect of being reunited with Appleton and the children once more. I dutifully reported to Sister Nivern's office – she was exactly the same. She sternly warned me about the growing laxity she'd witnessed in the nursing staff's observation of visiting hours.

'I am particularly concerned with a growing sense of over-familiarity with our patients and their parents,' Sister Skinflint told me. 'Strict rules of propriety are to be adhered